WOMEN AND REPRODUCTIVE TECHNOLOGIES

A sociological and historical study of the development of reproductive technologies, this book focuses on key technological developments through a biomedicalization lens with special attention to gender. Using *in vitro* fertilization (IVF) as a hub, it critically examines the main areas of related socio-technical developments: reproductive science, birth control, animal husbandry, genetics and reproductive medicine. Employing a critical framework to illuminate dominant discourses, the book also highlights examples of social resistance, as well as contradictory responses to new reproductive technologies. Over eight chapters, the author examines the social history of reproduction and sexuality, reproductive technologies from old to new and debates surrounding new reproductive technologies and genetic engineering. *Women and Reproductive Technologies* pays close attention to the interconnections between the business of reproduction (and replication industries), the sociality of reproduction (including reproductive justice) and what are considered the technologies themselves. As such, it constitutes essential reading for students and researchers in the fields of sociology, health studies and gender studies interested in the current state of human reproduction.

Annette Burfoot is Professor and Head of the Department of Sociology at Queen's University, Canada. She is the editor of *The Encyclopedia of Reproductive Technologies* and the four volume set *Visual Culture and Gender*, and the co-editor of *Killing Women: The Visual Culture of Gender and Violence*.

Derya Güngör received her PhD in Sociology from Queen's University in 2019. She is specialized in feminist theories, biopolitics, reproduction politics, pregnancy governance and sociology of medicine.

Routledge Research in Gender and Society

For more information about this series, please visit: https://www.routledge.com/Routledge-Research-in-Gender-and-Society/book-series/SE0271

WOMEN AND REPRODUCTIVE TECHNOLOGIES

The Socio-Economic Development of Technologies Changing the World

Annette Burfoot with Derya Güngör

Routledge
Taylor & Francis Group
LONDON AND NEW YORK

Cover image: Cherish Parrish (Ottawa/Pottawatomi), The Next Generation – Carriers of Culture, 2018, black ash and sweetgrass. Courtesy of the artist.

First published 2022
by Routledge
2 Park Square, Milton Park, Abingdon, Oxon OX14 4RN

and by Routledge
605 Third Avenue, New York, NY 10158

Routledge is an imprint of the Taylor & Francis Group, an informa business

British Library Cataloguing-in-Publication Data
A catalogue record for this book is available from the British Library

Library of Congress Cataloging-in-Publication Data
Names: Burfoot, Annette, author. | Güngör, Derya, author.
Title: Women and reproductive technologies: the socio-economic development of technologies changing the world / Annette Burfoot with Derya Güngör.
Description: Milton Park, Abingdon, Oxon; New York, NY: Routledge, 2022. | Series: Routledge research in gender and society | Includes bibliographical references and index.
Identifiers: LCCN 2021033897 (print) | LCCN 2021033898 (ebook) | ISBN 9781138606456 (hardback) | ISBN 9781138606463 (paperback) | ISBN 9780203772539 (ebook)
Subjects: LCSH: Human reproductive technology—Social aspects. | Women—Social conditions.
Classification: LCC RG133.5 .B87 2022 (print) | LCC RG133.5 (ebook) | DDC 362.1981/78—dc23
LC record available at https://lccn.loc.gov/2021033897
LC ebook record available at https://lccn.loc.gov/2021033898

ISBN: 9781138606456 (hbk)
ISBN: 9781138606463 (pbk)
ISBN: 9780429467646 (ebk)

DOI: 10.4324/9780429467646

Typeset in Bembo
by codeMantra

CONTENTS

ACKNOWLEDGEMENTS

Work of this kind is never done alone. I start at the beginning and thank Somer Brodribb who, over three decades ago, introduced me to Mary O'Brien and reproductive consciousness and to the possibility of thinking about things differently. This gave life to this project which reflects three decades of teaching a course on women and reproductive technology. Thanks to all the students over all those years who participated and helped me develop the ideas here. I am also grateful to the people at Queen's University who allowed me to research and write and provided me the opportunity to meet my colleague on this project, Dr. Derya Güngör. Derya was the midwife to this work and was present from its start. She was instrumental in the book's design and helped carry it to completion. I am grateful for the opportunity to work with this scholar of reproduction with such a steady and helpful hand.

Thanks to those at Routledge who helped carry this along from beginning to end. Neil Jordan was a calm, guiding hand from the proposal to submission, at which point Alice Salt capably took over.

Daily chats with my sister Nin also carried me along, especially as the pandemic hit and I had to juggle some pretty large balls in the air at home and at work. The laughter was priceless. A close circle of friends, Babi, Laura, Vicki and Tove, also helped to keep me sane and productive. Vicki, a lawyer, read through the chapter on legislation. And, finally, thanks to my domestic pod made up of my son Gabe and our dogs Hugo and Latte. The talks and walks made all the difference in the World! And maybe now I won't be so grumpy.

Any errors in this text are mine.

INTRODUCTION

When the birth of Louise Joy Brown was announced in 1978 as the world's first baby born from *in vitro* fertilization (IVF) or the world's first "test-tube baby," many took notice. There was fear that we were crossing a line into unmarked territory and exposing the human embryo like never before. What would happen to these children formed in cold glass containers in sterile labs? Would they be less human? Would they be monstrous? Would they die and feel it? This was science and medicine dealing with the most vulnerable stage of human becoming – should we really be messing about so? Many women, especially those of us in or near large modern cities and now used to routine medical attention to our reproductivity, saw this as further incursion. Not necessarily unwelcome, but was it necessary? Those critical of medical intervention into a normal part of human being continued to be critical and could see how genetic engineering would figure. However, more women who lived in poverty and social neglect with far less attention paid by modern medicine to their reproductivity didn't notice. Some religious authorities welcomed IVF as another step in promoting the reproduction of souls, while others sniffed the air and claimed the move too close to playing God. And a combination of all from the above worried over the status of the newly exposed human embryo.

The news heralded something very new, very important and a big change in how we handle reproduction. This book argues the opposite. Although the externalization of conception for the first time is significant and unique, the questions raised by the appearance of the first test-tube baby are not new, and neither are the motivations trailing behind. This was less a line suddenly crossed than a burst of success after many years of developments from various sectors – from animal husbandry to endocrinology. There are also systems at play combining biomedical financial interest, global geopolitics and evolving reproductive rights,

DOI: 10.4324/9780429467646-1

to name a few key ones. And throughout there are two important and increasingly overlooked constants: women's bodies or bodies that can conceive, gestate, birth and nurse are at the core, and socio-economic interests are always close to hand. How to make sense of it all?

Half of this text is devoted to developing an appreciation of the systems that scaffold what is typically understood as reproductive technology (when we add "technology" to the term we normally mean "new" reproductive technologies post-1978, Louise's birth year). The first four chapters examine ideas about reproduction as they change through the ages; the social, political and financial impacts of the modern medical age of reproduction; and our constant and shifting socio-economic controls of reproduction as well as sexuality. The second half of this book examines the nature of shifts in reproductive and genetic science and medicine beginning in the last quarter of the 20th century and examines them in terms of ongoing legislative challenges, the principles of reproductive justice and recent developments in the current systems of reproductivity and replication worldwide.

The first chapter examines key shifts in how we understand reproduction from veneration of the feminine reproductive to supposed genderless genetic recombination. It considers the major developments in reproductive thought, especially in terms of gender from the prehistoric times to today. There is an obvious decline in the valuation of the feminine reproductive over the ages, and a fast-rising sun starting mid-20th century and continuing into the 21st century in genetic replication. The current state of medicalization of reproduction and birth is explored in the second chapter as a logical development from centuries of denigration of feminine reproductivity and the recognition of value in the medical care of pregnancy and birth worldwide. The modern social control of reproductivity in terms of rights and social justice is the focus of Chapter 3, which covers various ways in which we as a society control the means of reproduction (access to conception and abortion) and how we recognize and limit family formation (kinship). This is explored further in the fourth chapter in terms of sexuality. Once we were able to distinguish between sexual desire and reproduction, significant sociopolitical developments in reproductive rights were achieved, allowing for both control over family size especially by women and the recognition of non-heterosexual communities and their rights which eventually included the right to reproduce. The commercial interest in the management of sexuality and reproduction is included.

Chapter 5 introduces the slate of the so-called new reproductive technologies and their constant companion, genetic engineering. Particular attention is played to the key characters involved in their development and how they link to a variety of fields including a well-established industry in dairy and meat, and growing speculation in genetic applications. Chapter 6 explores the difficult terrain of legislative response to new reproductive technology (NRT) applications in humans, including bringing under new legislation older reproductive technologies and initially hampering reproductive rights for single women and gay men. The challenge with legislating genetic science is also explored. In Chapter 7 we return to the issue of reproductive rights, but through an intersectional approach: reproductive justice. Here the focus is on access issues due to sexual orientation, global disparities and intranational racial and socio-economic inequalities. We examine feminist responses to NRTs along with responses by dominant religious authorities and growing LGBTQ2+ (lesbian, gay, bisexual, transgender, queer, two-spirited, plus others questioning their gender) communities giving voice to their sexual freedom and reproductive rights. The eighth and final chapter brings together many of the themes covered previously in the text by breaking down the meaning of each word in the phrase, women and new reproductive technology. In the conclusion, this analysis is extended into a selection of developments in NRTs and genetic engineering since 2010.

Throughout this volume concepts behind words such as woman, parent, right and technology are not seen as stable, nor are they untethered. The text is designed to draw attention to the variety of platforms on which reproduction occurs: the politics of kinship, gender discrimination and biomedicalized industries. It is hoped that after reading through this work you become aware of how far and deep reproduction and all of its issues spread. Also, we live in a time when we are about to take important steps into a world of replication; the more informed we are of how genetic engineering intersects with socio-economic systems, the better. This is one attempt.

1

REPRODUCTIVE THEORIES

Then and now

Our ideas of what reproduction is have changed over time. From the prehistoric to today, we have wrangled with the question, "where do babies come from?" Initially, we didn't understand the connection between sexual activity and reproduction. Then, once we thought we did, we became fascinated by (and restricted to) a male–female structure, with varying roles assigned to each gender, with the male normally coming out on top. This has extended to all of life in quests to explain the vibrant world around us – how does it keep going? How does reproduction vary between beings? Why and how do beings change over time? Can we control reproduction to our advantage? Should we? The 20th century is an important time in reproductive theory and practice: it marks not only the discovery and coding of an entire human genome (the genetic information unique to each human being), but also the achievement of almost 100% effective biochemical contraception and conception outside of the body. We have learned enough about reproduction and genetic replication to move human reproductive parts from one body to another, to freeze and store these parts and to examine and modify them genetically before bringing them to term. None of this would have been possible without what came beforehand in attempting to understand reproduction. Also, this is not a straight arrow of technical development and discovery, but more of a spiralling questioning often controlled by dominant interests where unexpected ideas from the distant past resurface and continue to play a part today.

The prehistoric veneration of a feminine divine

It is difficult to unearth the meaning of prehistoric imagery and artefact. We have little in the way of any recorded voice; only the images and sculpted pieces remain, usually in stone. However, especially throughout the 20th century, there

DOI: 10.4324/9780429467646-2

have been many attempts at making meaning of a growing collection of cave drawings and small stone figurines mostly from the Upper (or later) Paleolithic period (50000–10000 BCE or Before the Common Era, formerly BC or Before Christ). The Paleolithic period, defined by the presence of tools used by early humans, began over two and a half million years ago. These images and figurines have been considered through an archaeological lens in terms of possible meanings, belief systems and sociality. When searching the Internet for the Paleolithic era, a common figurine appears – the so-called Venus of Willendorf, a handheld, limestone figure of a rotund female with voluptuous breasts and buttocks, which was found in lower Austria, and is dated 30000–25000 BCE. Of course, the much later Roman goddess of beauty and love who shares this figurine's name is more commonly rendered in terms of heterosexual desire than venerated for feminine reproductivity, as is believed to be the case for these prehistoric figurines.

The European archaeologist, Marija Gimbutas, gathered, categorized and analysed over 2,000 images and figurines found mostly throughout Eastern Europe, from the Upper Paleolithic period, which is an era associated with the appearance of artefacts but before the development of agriculture (which occurred during the Neolithic period 10000–4500 BCE). She places the Venus figurine, and many like it, among a constellation of imagery focused on human female bodies, particularly their reproductive aspects. There are unabashed representations of vulvas, uteri and breasts, surrounded by and incorporating swirls, seeds and whirls that are believed to represent the cycle of life. Animals stand in for some of the venerated parts and reproductive functions: the hedgehog and the bull for the uterus, for example. Male figures also appear during this period but much more rarely, and typically as a protector of plants and animals or as consorts to the feminine figures. A host of historians and social scientists have mapped and attempted explanations of the reproductive female figures and images. Some, such as Gimbutas, describe a powerful social role for the feminine reproductive that dominates in prehistoric imaging: a venerated goddess.

Again, we do not know exactly how human reproduction was understood in prehistoric periods. We can imagine that given what people saw – a woman's body starting to swell at about the third month of pregnancy followed by the birth of a baby six months later, with nothing much obviously happening right after heterosexual copulation – the sexual activity was not associated with the reproductive outcome. Heterosexual sex was understood as separate from reproduction. There is ample evidence of reproduction being explained apart from heterosexual copulation, for example animal spirits or totems being associated with women's reproductivity. In about 3000 BCE, the bull, according to Gimbutas, was associated with reproducing women (and not with power of the thunder god as in later Indo-European mythology) because of the similarity between the bull's head and the female reproductive organs (the array of ovaries, fallopian tubes, ligaments and uterus). The hedgehog as prehistoric vessel is a representation of the human uterus (5000–4000 BCE).

The separation of coitus and birth allows for a female-centred philosophy of human reproduction where the feminine serves as a symbolic bridge between all life and its meaning and purpose. Bulging breasts, swollen bellies and exaggerated vulvas of the prehistoric human figurines are sometimes presented incised with concentric circles (read as the cyclical nature of life), while the head, a powerful symbol of the modern human being, is almost non-existent. By contemporary standards, these naked figures can be read as lewd, even pornographic. But those who contextualize the pieces historically and socially ignore the modern sexual triggers of the naked female body and focus attention on the meaning of reproduction-as-female. Some, like Gimbutas, argue that the imagery refers to how the female reproductive body was venerated for sustaining as well as explaining the prehistoric world.

Although the relatively very high number of prehistoric female figurines compared to male ones remains uncontested in modern archaeological studies (only 2–3% of the figurines unearthed are male), there has been a critical response to the female goddess theory. Important questions regarding contextualization and overgeneralization arise: How can you take so many varied figurines from a wide-ranging area, produced at various times, and make generalizations about a shared and singular significance among these figurines? The archaeologist, Richard Lesure, offers a method designed to "diffract" a single-goddess construct. He argues for a careful comparison of female figurines between areas – Mesoamerica and the Near East, and to not confuse how we make sense of the people producing the figurines and the symbols they use with the people themselves and their use of the images and figurines. This is sound advice for any historian and archaeologist. Indeed, this method does open up the figurines, and the people who made them and used them, to a much more detailed, contextualized and self-aware study. But such studies do not seem to be forthcoming. Lesure's caution also has the effect of distracting us from questions of why so many made the effort to create so many human female figurines, across great distances (the Near East, India, Mesoamerica and Europe), over thousands of years, always with feminine reproduction centrally featured alongside complex symbolism. And by comparison, there are virtually no human male figurines associated with reproduction. Why not?

There may be something of an explanation in Carl Liungman's – the Swedish scholar of symbols – description of the development of the symbol for Venus, which indicates both the planet and the Roman goddess (known as Aphrodite in Ancient Greece). The goddess Venus is represented by the symbol now meaning female in modern biological science (a small circle with a cross underneath), and meaning emancipated woman in the mid-20th century when the American-based women's liberation movement added a closed fist at the top of the cross within the circle. Clara Pinto-Correira credits Liungman with identifying an important shift in the meaning of Venus:

> The planet Venus, [female symbol], was in earlier times associated with a
> common goddess of fertility, war, sex and peace. This was true of nearly all

known ancient cultures around the Mediterranean. But from about 2400 until 250 B.C. this Venus goddess was gradually replaced by masculine divinities.

Enter the veneration of the male and masculinity, and what Riane Eisler, a cultural historian and evolutionary theorist, calls the "gylanic [gender equitable society]-androcratic [male dominant society] transformation." Hence the 20th-century addition of a clenched woman's fist to the symbol of Venus.

Ancient historic philosophies of generation: epigenesis

This transformation from societies where women's reproductivity was venerated to male-dominant societies occurs near the beginning of the historic age (defined by the arrival of writing in about 3200 BCE). In addition to text, early historic societies had cities and learning centres where philosophies of good government and ideal social life were argued and recorded, along with rationalizations of the world around them. Moving from artefacts and symbols to text, we get a better handle on what was thought about reproduction, especially from the classical Greek "father of philosophy," Aristotle (384–322 BCE). Although this is not the first example of writing on the meaning of reproduction, Aristotle's *Generation of Animals* is often referred to as one of the earliest theories of reproduction because of its detailed rationalization using a proto-scientific approach. It is interesting to note that the word "reproduction" was only coined in 1749 by the naturalist Georges-Louis Leclerc, Comte de Buffon (before then "generation" was the word commonly used). Aristotle made clear distinctions between gendered roles, which include assumed roles in his early scientific explanation of human reproduction. Aristotle distinguished between bloodless animals, chiefly insects (which were thought to reproduce spontaneously), and all the rest, including humans, which relied on distinct female and male contributions. Blood and heat purification played significant roles –probably drawn from prehistoric and pagan valuations of fire as both life-enhancing (providing heat in cold environments, cooking food, sealing and disinfecting wounds) and purifying (new life springs from burnt ground, healing elements can be distilled from boiled plant concoctions). Although this classical natural philosophy of human reproduction was somewhat empirical, it was limited to what could be seen by the human eye unaided by any magnification. At times there are elements in these theories based on pure conjecture, such as the role of female "semen."

By the time of Aristotle's work on human generation, a connection between heterosexual coitus and reproduction had been established: sex and reproduction were no longer separated. Autopsy practices of the day focused on genitalia: the womb, ovaries, the fallopian tubes (although not yet named so), the vagina, testicles and the penis, and the attached blood vessels (undifferentiated veins and arteries). Ovaries were understood as female versions of male testes. Sperm and eggs were not yet identified; only the fluids thought to carry reproductive components from both sexes were visible and figured in these theories of conception. The obvious absence of menstrual fluid once a woman became pregnant was read as the retention of that fluid to nourish the seed planted during the ejaculation of male semen. Both male and female reproductive fluids were thought to be generated from blood: male semen was understood as more distilled or perfect than female menstrual blood, which was more abundant but far less changed or perfected. Heat was the reason given for it. Men, the larger and stronger, and thus considered the more developed being, were argued by Aristotle to have a much greater ability to generate heat and perfect their blood into semen-as-seed. Women's role was to provide the place and nourishment for the male seed to grow. Important to note here is that this seed is not a preformed human being but acts on the material provided by the female (menstrual fluid as an inferior but necessary blood derivative) by providing a sort of formula or directions for embryonic development. This approach is known as epigenesis.

The historian of science, Nancy Tuana, reminds us of Aristotle's description of male ejaculate as "the principle of soul," which also elevates the male role in reproduction to a spiritual level, leaving the female one as mundane (meaning literally, of the world) and "just a nurse to the seed." This view did not exactly match other classical theorists, including Hippocrates (c460–370 BCE), who believed that a foetus resulted from a combination of male and female semen, albeit the female version being invisible and weaker than that of the male. The Greek physician, surgeon and natural philosopher Galen (130–210 AD), who is often cited as one of the founders of modern medicine, initially embraced Hippocrates' notion that female and male semen combined to form the embryo. However, without the ability to visualize female semen, Galen eventually adopted Aristotle's theory of generation that reduced the female role to a passive and inferior one, explaining how the internalization of female genitalia was a sign of how a lack of heat in the female means that the genitalia does not fully unfold or bloom outwards as male genitalia. The theory of the superior male role in reproduction is perpetuated for over a 1,000 years: Saint Gregory of Nyssa (335–394 AD) argues that the embryo is implanted in the female by the male; Saint Thomas Aquinas (1225–1274) argues that only God can produce form in matter, so "the active seminal power" of man's seed acts as a medium between God and mankind; and the Judaic *Midrash Rabbah Genesis* (1545) repeats Aristotle's theory that the male sperm acts upon the female matter (menses) to give it form.

Reproductive theory then moves to establish what Tuana calls the "anatomical tradition" which, alongside natural philosophies of reproduction, helps spread the word. The 1575 illustrations of incorrect penis- and testes-shaped female genitalia attributed to the work of German surgeon von Georg Bartisch indicate female reproductive anatomy as a version of the male. The Belgian physician and "father of modern anatomy," Andreas Vesalius (1514–1564), in his five-volume illustration of the human body, *De Humani Corpus Fabrica*, shows an anatomically incorrect image of the ovaries that is used to distinguish between a hot ovary and a cool one based on the blood supply and to address Galen's criticism of Aristotle's theory of generation as incomplete. Vesalius' images attempt to prove how the "natural deficiency" of the female is reproduced in human reproduction: female foetuses are generated from the left ovary thought to be fed by cooler, unpurified blood; males are generated from the right ovary thought to be served by a hotter, purified blood supply. Actually these early anatomists mixed up the functions of ovarian veins (which take blood away from the ovary) and arteries (which bring blood to the ovary); but human anatomy in this period is such that the slight difference between left and right vein attachment to the ovaries rationalized the discriminatory theory of sexual difference. Thanks to inexpensive 16th-century printing techniques, images from the *Fabrica* became widely available and well known, and so we arrive at the onset of the Scientific Revolution with women's "natural inferiority" to men well established and based on broadly accepted, discriminatory theories of sexually determined reproductive capacities.

The scientific revolution and preformationism

This gender discrimination, that embryos develop gradually from unorganized matter into the perfect human form, with the male seed as the activating agent and the female as passive nurturer, persisted over 1,200 years. With advancements starting in the 1600s in anatomy, especially microscopic-aided examination, and the development of scientific thought and method in general, things begin to change in the world of human reproductive theory. William Harvey (1578–1657), a renowned British physician and scientist, took up the work of Hippocrates and Aristotle on the generation of animals, and at the end of his career made an unsubstantiated claim that female eggs played a significant role in reproduction: *ex ovo omne vivum* (every living thing comes from an egg). This is not surprising, given that since classical Greece, those interested in explaining reproduction often examined chicken eggs and embryos. However, Harvey could not find any sign of eggs in the mammals he examined and concluded that reproduction occurred in the uterus following coitus with a combination of difficult-to-determine male and female contributions, but he continued to assert that nothing substantive came from the female "testes" (ovaries). The medical historian, Mathew Cobb, calls our attention to this period and focuses on the 1660s–1670s, shortly after Harvey's statement about the significance of eggs, when evidence appears of human egg function (not yet of the egg itself) soon followed by the visual discovery of sperm.

Typical of the time, gentlemen scientists with little training and education provided the means and incentives for scientific exploration. One such gentleman who was once a French ambassador, Melchisedec Thévenot, brought two medical students from Leiden University to his home in Paris to explore the generation of animals. The students, Jan Swammerdam and Niels Stenson (known as Steno), were struck with the task of disproving Rene Descartes' theoretical approach to generation that followed Aristotle's, using the emerging scientific method based on empirical evidence and replicable experimentation. Although neither student found anything during their stay with Thévenot, they became motivated to continue with the work on their own. Because Swammerdam was primarily interested in insects, he was the first to state, with empirical evidence, that insects were neither bloodless nor did they spontaneously generate but reproduced with eggs. In 1669, like Harvey, he claimed boldly, "all animals come from an egg laid by a female of the same species." This theory, known as ovism, challenged almost 2000 years of thought that animals generated either spontaneously or with little female agency. Steno made a similar claim comparing the reproductive tracts of egg-laying rays, dogfish that give birth to live young, to women and sheep. Because of the similarities between them he concluded that eggs must be present in all these animals, whether they are mammals or not. Swammerdam looked for eggs in the ovaries of dead women and competed with a student colleague, Renier de Graaf, to be the first to prove they exist. Relying on dissected rabbit ovaries, de Graaf published in 1672 a new treatise on the generative organs of women (*De Mulierum Organis Generationi Inservientibus Tractatus Novus*) and argued that the follicles (raised bumps) visible on rabbits' ovaries were eggs (which is why we now refer to ovarian follicles as Graafian follicles). De Graaf pointed out in his treatise that Steno had claimed that ovaries contained eggs, but he could not see them. Nor could de Graaf, but he was able to prove their existence through their function using the new scientific method of empirical experimentation. He proved that the follicles (eggs) moved from the ovary to the fallopian tubes (described previously by Gabriele Fallopius, 1523–1562). In rabbits he saw small spherical shapes (fertilized eggs) appear in the tubes following sexual intercourse and noted that their number never exceeded the number of ovarian follicles found in the same animal just before the sexual activity. Without the identification of sperm, and unable to find traces of semen in the tubes, de Graaf concluded that a male "vapour" fertilized the eggs.

Also typical of the Scientific Revolution is the establishment of societies of scientists as a means of professionalizing and disseminating the growing scientific experimental work. These societies were found in most western European countries and became powerful and influential. Among the most influential is the British Royal Society of London for Improving Natural Knowledge (commonly referred to as the Royal Society), which was established in 1660 and continues today. The Royal Society reviewed and published the so-called discoveries, many of which involved the new scientific instrument, the microscope. In his submission of his work to the Royal Society, de Graaf mentioned the work of his friend, a draper in Delft, Antonie van Leeuwenhoek (1632–1723), who taught himself how to grind lenses, made a particularly powerful microscope and began observing with it. Although not a trained scientist, Leeuwenhoek and the Royal Society enjoyed a 50-year relationship, and his simple but effective microscope design was distributed throughout the Dutch Republic to become a powerful aid to the new scientific method enjoyed by many gentlemen. Swammerdam was among those who relied on the easy-to-use, single-lens microscope and used it to draw the first images of initial cell divisions in a fertilized frog egg. Medical illustration that had long been based on gross anatomy (that visible to the naked eye) moved to the microscopic.

The microscope allowed for the exploration of a new tiny terrain that became the focus of reproductive theory between the late 17th and mid-19th centuries. When Leeuwenhoek came across millions of little "animalcules" swimming in his own semen (which he called *spermatozoa* or sperm animals), a new and energetic character entered the stage of reproductive theory, ready to address the matter of how the male reproductive contribution occurred in concrete and demonstrable terms. Initially the function of these animalcules was not understood; in fact, Leeuwenhoek argued that other matter in the semen which he saw under his microscope (tiny vessels) was more interesting and concluded (with no evidence, and reverting to Aristotle's theoretical position) that, "it is exclusively the male semen that forms the foetus and that all the woman may contribute only serves to receive the semen and feed it." Although credited with the discovery of sperm, it was not Leeuwenhoek who recognized their function in reproduction. Despite the delay in publication of Leeuwenhoek's discovery of sperm in semen, word got out, and others began examining semen through their own microscopes and found "little worms" in dog and mice semen. The Dutch physicist, Christaan Huygens (1629–1695), published in 1678 that these findings were "extremely important and will provide material for those who seriously study the generation of animals," which it did.

The human egg, which is much larger than a sperm but more difficult to access, was not identified until 1827 by Karl Ernst von Baer. It took another half century to put forward a theory of reproduction based on the fusion of the egg and sperm, which was made by Oscar Hertwig. Meanwhile, over 150 years during the 17th and 18th centuries, reproductive theorists continued to speculate on the meaning of the microscopic visions in terms of preformed beings, with emphasis either on the female egg (ovists) or the male sperm (spermists). Preformationists marked a significant move away from the earlier epigenecists – from Aristotle to Harvey – and believed the entire entity of a being was contained in its generative seed; it just required the correct conditions for unfolding or development.

As the Scientific Revolution heralded a new way of seeing the world, and especially of determining what constituted the truth about the world, this did not mean that well-developed religious truths and their explanations for how and why we exist suddenly disappeared. For centuries, religious and early scientific belief systems worked together. What Pinto-Correia calls "programmed encasement" or the Russian doll metaphor refers to a long-standing human fascination with a hierarchy of mysteries, or the box hidden in another box which is hidden in another box, and so on. According to Christian belief, the primary creator, God, is everywhere and always waiting to be revealed according to His plan. The knowledge of God is mysterious and has to be earned. The struggle between early theories of reproduction, epigenesis versus preformation, demonstrates a similar quest to open reproductive mysteries to human understanding (and eventually control). Both of these sets of concealed mysteries, especially those explaining creation, can be linked to the prehistoric spirals signifying (think some) the circularity of life. However, the more modern explanations, both religious and secular, are mechanistic and one way, not circular, and are driven by a desire to know the origin and author of all generation with infinities of scale stretching in both directions from our key reference point, the human being: downwards and inside to the microscopic, and outside and upwards towards the astronomical heavens and the beginning of it all.

Modern reproductive science: genetic recombination

As modern science was developing, so were philosophies of knowledge and being (commonly referred to as the Age of Enlightenment-1685–1815), all alongside accepted religious beliefs of the time. There are two important streams of thought here that relate to the preformation theory of generation, which was dominant at the time: Man is a being of reason where reason is God, but man is free to make reasonable meaning of the universe (represented by the French philosopher and mathematician, Rene Descartes-1596–1650, who is often quoted as saying, "I think, therefore I am"). The second stream sees man as constantly striving to understand God's complex and ungraspable mechanistic universe or boxes within boxes (represented by the English mathematician, physicist and theologian Isaac Newton, 1643–1727; and the French philosopher and historian Voltaire,1694–1778). It is the latter stream of thought that is associated with the preformation theory of reproduction that dominates during the Enlightenment period.

Perhaps because early seed theories came very close to atheism when they argued that some form of male agent acted upon disorganized female matter to give rise to human form, preformationists, whether focused on the role of the egg or the sperm, believed the entire form was already contained in the germ or seed of reproduction. As Pinta-Correia puts it, the battle between the preformationists was focused on "where God had encased all organisms destined to come to come to life on earth: the egg [or] the spermatozoan." Although preformationist theory briefly provided a more active role for the female contribution to human reproduction than had been seen for millennia, the female reproductive role remained restricted by persistent beliefs in the superiority of the male role in procreation, heavily influenced by theological beliefs in masculine origins generally.

By the start of the 20th century, the profession of scientists and physicians was well established through expanding systems of public and higher education. Reproduction theory was housed in new disciplines including evolutionary and cell biology, embryology and gynecology. Cells were first seen in 1665 under the microscope and identified by the British scientist, Robert Hooke, who thought what he saw were like the monks' cells in a monastery. With the development of more powerful microscopes, cell components and functions were observed and gave rise to cell theory, which was formulated and credited to Matthias Schleiden and Theodor Schwann in 1839. This signalled the end of preformationism, as well as theories of spontaneous generation. Instead, cell theory claimed that these newly discovered entities regenerate through division (*Omnis cellula e cellula*) and are the basis, in terms of both structure and function, of all organisms. This allowed for the "animalcules" and "follicles" first detected by 17th-century eyes to be understood in new terms: cellular parts of a complex reproductive functional system.

And then came the gene. In *The Fundamentals of Genetics* by Leslie Vega and Bret White we learn that inheritance of attributes had long been observed: herders and others dealing with domesticated animals watched as traits passed from one animal to its progeny, and farmers understood the same happened in plants. And these traits could be controlled through breeding practices such as those developed in a proto-scientific manner by the British agriculturalist, Robert Bakewell, who, in the mid-18th century, separated his male and female livestock to control their inter-breeding for desirable traits and against non-desirable ones. Meanwhile, in the developing profession of medicine, physicians were observing how diseases were passed from one family member to another: Down's syndrome was described in 1866. At the same time, Gregor Mendel, an Augustinian friar and scientist who is now acknowledged as the "founder of modern genetics," studied the inherited traits of peas and discovered recessive and dominant inherited traits. Charles Darwin published *The Origin of Species* in 1859, where he outlined the theory of how inherited traits change over time or evolve, which holds today. All of these developments expanded theories of human reproduction by extending our understanding of the function of reproduction. The newly identified egg and sperm cells combined to create a new organism, and in doing so, they carried forward traits (including those associated with visual appearance and disease), and then they recombined to give rise to new traits allowing the organism to change over time, or evolve. One species can even develop into another called "pangenesis," from which the word gene is derived. Once again, we are drawn into profound questions of who we are, from where we come, and who we will become, but now outside of religious terms.

The chromosome or "coloured body" is a thread-like structure within cells containing DNA and proteins but was not initially understood in such detail. The chromosome was first seen in the early 19th century by several scientists and with new dying techniques, was detailed in terms of structure and function (mitosis or cell division producing two identical daughter cells) by the German anatomist Walther Flemming in 1882. However, Flemming did not know of Mendel's earlier work on the theory and mechanics of inheritance in plants and made no links between the chromosome and heredity. In 1868, a weak acid in white blood cells was discovered, which we now know as DNA, and in 1889 the Dutch botanist, Hugo de Vries, argued that "inheritance of specific traits in organisms comes in particles... [called] (pan)genes." In the early 20th century, chromosomes were seen to be heredity units and necessary for embryonic development. Then genetic discoveries started to tumble forward: A genetic map of a chromosome was first made in 1913, and sex-linked inheritance was discovered. Between the 1930s and 1950s, distinctive contributions were identified for the cell nucleus (where DNA was discovered) and its surrounding material, called cytoplasm (where RNA was identified). At the same time, the "crossing over" or interchange of genetic material between two different chromosomes as the cause of recombination was demonstrated by American cell geneticists Barbara McClintock and Harriet Creighton. As the Second World War came to a close, DNA was isolated as the genetic material responsible for cellular transformation, and shortly afterwards the main components of DNA, nitrogenous bases or guanine (G), adenine (A), cytosine (C) and thymine (T), were found to be always present in equal proportions to each other, and paired: GA and CT. An X-ray image of DNA was made in 1952, and a year later the combined work of British molecular biologist Francis Crick and X-ray crystallographer Rosalind Franklin, with the American molecular biologist James Watson, described the DNA as a double helix structure. In 1955, the American cell geneticist, Joe Hin Tjio, determined the number of chromosomes in humans to be 46, as the mechanics of cellular division and the distribution of chromosomes from parents to offspring was clarified. We have arrived at the theory of reproduction as equal genetic contributions from both parents that recombine to produce a genetically distinct being. Genesis is genetic.

To be precise, these developments are understood as epigenetic as with Aristotle's theory of generation. But where Aristotle thought that the undifferentiated essence of being (seed) was passed from the male to the female to be nourished and formed into a human being, contemporary epigenesis focuses on the differentiation of cells from undifferentiated cells with equal male and female genetic contributions. Twentieth-century theories of reproduction continued to focus on the mechanics of cellular genetic differentiation and have resulted in the engineering of reproduction and genetic replication. In principle, farmers controlling for desired traits in animals and plants over centuries were early genetic engineers: penning animals to control their mating controlled the expression and recombination of their genes. This took time, however, and was hit-or-miss in securing desirable traits and avoiding undesirable ones. As microscopes grew more powerful and micro manipulation machines and biochemical instruments allowed for scientists to not only identify and move cells but to strip cells down to their functional components, a much quicker and more precise manipulation of genetic traits evolved.

In terms of reproductive theories and the explosion of scientific research throughout the 20th century, reproduction was not reduced to only genetic recombination. Again, based on what could be seen, the initial understanding of beings as powered machines in the 19th century focused on the complex array of nerves found throughout the body and attached to almost everything visible: organs (including ovaries and testes) and muscles. The historian of medicine and science, Chandak Sengoopta, describes this as the "neural model" of human being which included reproduction (and inspired the story of Frankenstein). But in the early 20th century, this model quickly gave way to hormones as not only agents and anti-agents in the reproductive process, but also as leading actors in emerging theories of human *in utero* development. After cutting up gonads in rabbits and guinea pigs, and re-implanting them away from nerves, scientists discovered that something other than nerves activated growth and change. Endocrine (hormonal) gland organs, including the gonads (ovaries and testes), were found to excrete a fluid that was not blood but was released into and carried by the blood. In 1905, the British physiologist Ernest Starling named these excretions "hormones" after the Greek word for excitement or arousal; hormones were identified as a biochemical agent that can make change, like nerves and their innervation power.

Undetermined hormones were valued and used crudely in medical practice from the mid-19th century as a sort of rejuvenating tonic with the potency to excite or depress sexual development and behaviour. In the late 19th century, especially in France, gonads were being removed from slaughtered animals, dried, ground up and administered as the medical practice of "organotherapy." This so-called treatment was clearly sexed and problematic from the start: male gonadal derivatives were used in men in an attempt to reverse impotence and senility, while female gonadal derivatives were used in women for uterine disorders (heavy bleeding) and hysteria (which literally means wandering womb).

A woman's reproductive capacity was often associated with her mental health at this time and was a common rationale for preventing women from participating in the public world (such as attending university and practising as a doctor or lawyer) as it would overtax their brains, and thus hamper their natural reproductive role. Aside from organotherapy, the removal of a woman's ovaries began in 1872 in Germany as a treatment for "menstrual madness," nymphomania, masturbation and hysteria, among other female ailments. Ovariectomies were practised liberally by physicians throughout western Europe until after the First World War. Besides being a highly questionable medical practice, this generated a significant and valuable source of human ovaries and ovarian tissue for research, medical practice and the distillation of hormones for pharmaceutical use. It also helped provide the rationale for the medicalization of female reproduction as it contributed to a new and growing industry in hormones.

The Dutch social scientist Nelly Oudshoorn provides an important and critical overview of the making of sex hormones. Initially sex hormones were derived from organs in animals used in food production, and in 1923, the German Physician Ernst Laqueur signed a contract with a Dutch slaughterhouse to secure access to organ products to be processed for medical and scientific use. After sex hormones were later sourced in urine (horses', and then pregnant women's), Laqueur created the world-renowned hormone pharmaceutical company, Organon, a key player in the development of human *in vitro* fertilization (IVF).

The discrimination in sourcing for sex hormones was perpetuated by medical, scientific and pharmaceutical practices in the early 20th century, from whole organ or gland treatments to ones based on biochemicals distilled from the glands.

The need for testing for the presence of specific hormones and the ability to distill them out of source material (for example, urine) gave rise to a profession of biochemists and to an adjunct industry of hormone assays (or testing), which resulted in the pregnancy test made accessible to women on a do-it-yourself basis by the inventor and graphic designer Meg Crane in 1967. Crane worked for Organon at the time. Oudshoorn argues that the struggle for access to and control over the distribution of newly discovered sex hormones resulted in a disproportionate focus on female sex hormones, female fertility and female reproductivity. This was partly due to difficulties in sourcing male sex hormones because of physiological factors: sex hormone in men's urine is very weak compared to that in pregnant women's urine. Another part has to do with scientific and medical fascinations with the ovary and its role in reproduction established in the 19th century, which provided ample reasons and opportunities for collecting female sex hormones. Also, during this period, women were increasingly medicalized because of their reproductivity and because of perceived links between an actively reproductive female and her overall well-being, which included meeting requirements of social feminine norms. Women were literally more available to study, in whole or in their parts, and there was more reason to do so furnished both by professional authorities in science and medicine and from pressures stemming from social expectations regarding women's primary role in society as a reproducing being.

The emphasis between 1929 and 1935 on studying various glands and their hormonal secretions led to what the physiologist Alan Parkes called "the heroic age of reproductive endocrinology." A much clearer picture of the reproductive hormonal dance or "orchestra" involved in maturing and releasing the egg (follicle stimulating hormone or FSH and luteinizing hormone or LH), readying it for fertilization and preparing the uterine wall for implantation of the fertilized egg (oestrogen and progesterone), emerged at this time. The bisexuality of sex hormones was discovered: both men and women produce both types of sex hormones; it is a question of balance as to what sexual trait is expressed. And finally, the role of the brain was described, particularly hormonal messaging between the ovaries, the pituitary gland and the hypothalamus.

Oudshoorn indicates how, initially, these discoveries led to various medical applications of gonadal-based hormones including the treatment of senility and hemophilia with oestrogen derived from sheep placentas and ovaries. Also, a connection between sex hormones, especially oestrogen, and some cancers was suspected. The "most secret quintessence of life," or the male hormone androgen, was distilled in 1931 with great effort from 25,000 litres of male urine in Germany by the chemist Adolf Butenandt and was renamed by Laqueur in 1935 (with research funding by Organon) as "testosterone." Its medical application induced increased muscle mass and hair growth and was used to treat symptoms of ageing in men (called the "male climacteric" or a form of male menopause) including senility and declining sexual function, but with disappointing results in otherwise normal men. As hormones became associated with behaviour, oestrogen was used in women diagnosed with an array of now questionable mental illnesses, including hysteria. Testosterone was used to "treat" male homosexuality (female homosexuality went largely unrecognized in the early 20th century and escaped such attention). In a period where gender was considered distinct, even oppositional, in terms of physicality and behaviour, hormones held out the promise to normalize perceived abnormalities or imbalances in both, and thus to stabilize the social and moral norms of the sexually conservative Victorian age.

Sengoopta explains how the distinction between male and female sex hormones was complex, and sometimes misguided. The German physician, homosexual activist and founder of the Berlin Institute for Sexual Science, Magnus Hirschfeld, put forward the "principle of universal sexual intermediacy" as an indication that all people contained a balance of male and female factors, physical and mental, and sometimes that balance failed. His Austrian colleague, the physiologist Eugen Steinach, began studying the basis of sexual difference in 1912. He found the feminization of males possible through castration, and to a far lesser degree, the masculinization of women through castration and testicular transplant. This led initially to a very financially successful phase of vasectomy in older men as an anti-ageing and virilizing treatment (it was thought to trigger the pituitary gland and its growth hormone). A similar technique was tried in women shortly afterwards using the heating and radiation of the ovaries and was considered successful in terms of "rejuvenating" post-menopausal females. These techniques relied on the 1920s discovery by Harvey Cushing of the function of the tiny pituitary gland lying deep at the base of the brain, "like the nugget in the innermost series of Chinese boxes," as the ignition for all glandular secretions including the ovaries and testes, and was considered a fountain of youth. However, using sex hormones to control fertility remained out of reach in the first half of the 20th century. With oestrogen alone, physicians could not trigger menstruation in a woman unable to menstruate, but it was discovered that a combination of progestin (considered a male sex hormone) and oestrogen would lead to the complex build-up of the blood-filled lining of the uterus required to nourish the fertilized egg if present, and to be released as menstrual fluid if not.

Meanwhile, what Sengoopta calls "an ever-expanding cast of new characters" entered the scene of human reproduction. The adrenal glands (sitting atop each kidney and the source of the hormone adrenaline) became known during the early part of the 20th century as significant players in human development. A sexual component of the gland, "the third gonad," was described in the 1950s and was held responsible for "virilizing" women and was even blamed for the earlier Suffragette movement! The pineal gland (found in the brain and now known as the source of the hormone melatonin used to regulate sleep) was thought to cause premature sexual behaviour in children. In the 1930s, the thymus gland found in the upper chest (the source of T cells and most active in pre-adolescents in establishing the immune system) was suspected of playing a role in the hormone or endocrine system that was then understood to orchestrate growth, including sexual maturation and reproduction. And king among these was considered the pituitary gland, which in 1935 Bernhard Zondek called "the motor of all endocrine function." As was becoming a common cycle, initially surgery, in this case pituitary transplants, was used to treat growth and development disorders. Once growth hormones or gonadotrophins were identified and distilled, they were used in treatment, but not yet effectively for infertility, even though this higher level of hormone signalling was known to influence the sexual gonads (ovaries and testes). Also, despite early endocrinology recognizing that sex hormones were not sexually exclusive, women and men both produced and required so-called female and male sex hormones, sex hormones remain tightly associated with gendered traits today.

The mid-20th century brought important developments in understanding the complex combination of biochemical and neurobiological aspects of reproduction. Although the "era of the glands" in the early part of the century focused there, it came after a considerable time of early scientific exploration of the neurological system as an electric generator of growth and development. In the early part of the 19th century Giovanni Aldini and Alessandro Volta were at odds over the role of "animal electricity" as potential reanimation. It was fairly widely known that applying electrical current through the system of nerves could stimulate muscular movement in dead animals and cadavers. Could applying this life force not bring them back to life? It was these proto-neurological experiments and debates about life forces that inspired Mary Shelley's *Frankenstein* in 1818. And they were not forgotten a century later as hormones entered the scene as life stimulators: in the mid-1930s, the biologist Francis Marshall demonstrated how electrically stimulating a rabbit's head encouraged ovulation. By the mid-20th century, the link between the brain and the glands was described as a feedback circuit looping between the hypothalamus (a small region of the brain responsible for signalling the release of hormones), the pituitary gland and the sexual gonadal glands. It was not simply the presence of hormones that was important to human reproduction, but when they appeared and where, in what quantity, in which combination – all of this in concert with neural messaging. Also, electrical stimulation continues to play a significant part in reproductivity and is a key to several IVF-based techniques and some aspects of genetic engineering of the embryo.

Perhaps one of the most significant applications stemming from these advances in hormones, the neural system and reproductivity was the oral contraceptive, the Pill. The Pill was developed in the mid-20th century by American endocrine scientists Gregory Pincus and Min Chueh Chang and the gynaecologist John Rock, and received crucial funding support from the American heiress Katherine Dexter McCormick at the urging of her friend, the birth control advocate Margaret Sanger. Sanger opened the first American birth control clinic in 1916; the Pill was approved for clinical use in 1957. This progress in controlling reproductive hormones represents what sociologists of science such as Celia Roberts characterize as a sociobiological shift. It was not simply new insights into the workings of reproductive hormones that led to the Pill's development, but the constant demand, especially by women, for an effective means of controlling their reproduction. Its application resulted in material changes to women's bodies and lives, as well as to the nature of the social body around the world. And it was a nascent social movement that connected women's control of their reproductivity with social well-being that drove this significant development of scientific understanding and medical applications within reproduction.

Biochemists came a long way in identifying and distilling an array of hormones required to generate sperm and mature eggs and to prepare the uterus for implantation, but they needed to perfect the synthesis of these hormones in order to manipulate them and to provide effective treatment. Besides a highly effective oral contraceptive, some key medical applications of hormones in the mid-20th century included the treatment of diabetes with the hormone insulin and the treatment of dwarfism with human growth hormone. Early on there were some attempts at treating male and female infertility with doses of male and female hormones, respectively, with measurable success with the latter, but the picture was not clear as to what exactly was happening in the reproductive neuro-endocrine system. This would require the developments that led to IVF in humans in the early 1980s.

Assisted reproduction and genetic replication

Theories of reproduction in the early 20th century depended on an intense triangulation of lab-based technical expertise (such as the emerging profession of biochemists), animal husbandry (for ample and steady supplies of organs and glands for hormones and sometimes for research subjects) and medical practice (particularly gynaecology and obstetrics). The same was true with the engineering of human reproduction, including genetics, as key areas of development in reproductive theory in the later 20th century and early 21st century. The shift was signalled by the externalization of human conception from the body known as IVF. Key players in this area of reproductive theoretical development included pharmacy companies (commercial interest spurring developments in hormone manufacture and hormonal screening), medical practice (chiefly in the new sub-specialties of assisted reproductive technologies and reproductive medicine), lab-based technicians (for gamete preparation and storage), scientists (geneticists and developmental biologists keen to access human gametes and cellular embryos for experimentation) and veterinarian science (alongside animal husbandry it provided support to develop breeding techniques associated with burgeoning food industries in meat and dairy).

During the latter half of the 20th century, key developments in reproductive theory included a refinement in the understanding of the complex system of hormones, organs, neural signalling and genetic exchange. These theoretical developments gave way to techniques that allowed for control of key aspects of the reproductive process at the moment of conception, such as developing a medium or nutritional fluid to support gametes and very young embryos outside of the body. Hormonal ovarian stimulation was mastered to produce more than a single egg each cycle. The freezing and storage of gametes and embryos was achieved. Hormonal enhancements generated higher rates of success with embryo implantation and allowed for embryo donation and surrogate pregnancy. Methods for genetic screening and the manipulation of pre implanted embryos were also developed.

These technical procedures in the handling of reproductive components and processes were honed chiefly in non-human applications first. The ability to transfer embryos came from initial attempts with rabbits, especially by the British zoologist and embryologist Walter Heape. The lab work at the turn of the 20th century exploring embryology, glands and their effects on growth and sex attributes was quickly taken up in animal husbandry as a way of controlling for desired genetic traits in animals that served the food industry. For example, it was more efficient to transfer embryos from a cow with high milk fat content into hormonally readied surrogate cows to bring the desired embryos to term than wait out the ten-month gestation period in the cow each time she became pregnant before being able to start another reproductive cycle. By flushing out the desired embryos at an early stage of pregnancy and implanting them in surrogates, you could have several cows pregnant at the same time with the desired genetic traits. Techniques of sperm donation, sperm management (including freezing) and artificial insemination were well established when cow, sheep and pig embryo flushing and transfer became successful in the 1950s, although only fresh embryos at this point were used (transported in live rabbits) as embryo freezing was not yet possible. Oocyte or egg freezing was far trickier and, unlike with the storing of sperm and embryos, egg freezing entered routine medical practice much later in the early 2000s, almost half a century after success in sperm freezing, and 25 years after embryo freezing. By 2010, more had been learned about the egg's membrane or covering and cellular susceptibility to breaking up when frozen and thawed. Also, at this time reproductive scientists figured out how to maintain the cell's structural and genetic integrity with particular freezing agents and a quick-freezing process.

The reproductive physiologist Martin Johnson provides a useful overview of the key developments in IVF techniques that advanced knowledge of reproduction include the development of culture media in which to keep and nourish eggs and newly formed embryos outside of the body (the same in sperm management had developed much earlier). Initially, during the late 1960s, chiefly mouse eggs and embryos were kept alive and encouraged to continue development in blood or serum-based media, sometimes with the addition of fallopian tube cells, or placed in parts of the tubes themselves. Experiments with culturing human eggs outside of the body started in 1944 and proceeded with experimentations using human and fetal calf serum, the patient's own serum, amniotic fluid and fallopian tubes. They also experimented throughout the 1980s and the early 1990s with a variety of cell lines (differentiated cells distilled from various parts of bodies and kept alive and replicating) variously combined, and then moved to a "back-to-nature strategy" in the late 1990s and early 2000s. What was learned as a result of this considerable experimentation, crucial to the success of IVF as a safe medical application, was that the naturally occurring environment for eggs and embryos is complex, and it changes as the process of fertilization progresses over time and in place, for example, levels of lactate and glucose (nourishment for early forming embryos) in the fallopian tubes and uterus change as the fertilized egg and embryo's needs change. Thanks to increased understanding of cells and genetics, we now know that sex cells (eggs and sperm) and early forming embryos go through "precisely orchestrated events" of division and genetic activation that, without proper support (such as culture media), could have serious effects on the outcome of implantation and, more importantly, on the formation of the being.

Robert Edwards was the British physiologist credited, along with the British gynaecologist Patrick Steptoe, with the first successful human IVF and as a pioneer of modern assisted reproduction. Edward's 1955 PhD thesis focused on ways of creating genetic abnormalities in mammalian (mice) eggs in the hope of developing applications in animal breeding and to further knowledge about genetic development. In particular, Edwards' work built on the knowledge of cell parts called centrioles, which were observed in the late 1800s and whose function in genetic replication was described in the 1950s.

During the latter part of the 20th century and into the 21st, the significant developments in reproductive theory were largely genetic based. This meant a turn away from the relatively large-scale realm of gonads – ovaries and testes – and their respective sex cells – eggs and sperm – to the genetic helix. The reproductive organs and their complex hormonal interplay became infrastructure and stages in a very promising world where the essence of what makes us human was understood as a code. This code not only opened doors to understanding the expression of genetic traits but shifted reproductive theory to theories of replication. Earlier developments in biochemistry and cellular biology came to play in describing the human genome and its function. The genome, unique to each being from plant to human, is made up of a molecule which has a spiralling ladder-like structure (the double helix) known as DNA (deoxyribonucleic acid) that can be unzipped up the middle and zipped up again. Each side of each rung of the ladder is made up of one of the four possible bases, known as the building blocks of DNA: A, G, C and T (used cleverly to title the film about genetic engineering, *Gattaca*). Although the Swiss physician and biologist Friedrich Miescher isolated DNA in 1869, its molecular structure and function was described in 1953 by Watson and Crick, with Franklin's support. DNA clusters around proteins in the cell forming chromosomes. Humans have 23 chromosome pairs in each cell (46 in total); 22 of these pairs look the same in males and female; one pair, the sex chromosome, is different. In males it is an X and Y chromosome pair, and in females two X chromosomes are paired. During reproduction it was learned, in part thanks to the key Meselson-Stahl experiment (1953–1957), that the DNA from each parent's sex chromosomes (eggs and sperm in animals) unzip, the half ladder (DNA strand or single helix) of each parent meets and zips up to form a new DNA or ladder and a distinct genetically coded being. This is why we carry some traits of our mother and some of our father. This process of unzipping and zipping up with a different side of the ladder is widely regarded as the basis of contemporary reproductive biology. DNA with its coding structure is commonly characterized as "the blueprint" of life or as argued by the anthropologist Sarah Franklin as "life itself," and what the social scientist, Joan Fujimura calls, "vital signs."

Also important to contemporary reproductive theory is what happens when things go wrong along the length of the helix or ladder. DNA working with another acid molecule, RNA, instructs cells on how to form. It does this with packets of information or genes, which are a series of rungs on the ladder that are coded to produce a specific protein. Keep in mind that every human genome has about 3 million base pairs (rungs), which are contained in each cell of the body (divided between the 23 chromosomes). If you stretched one cell's DNA (ladders) out they would be about two meters long. All of the DNA in one person stretched out end to end would be about twice the diameter of the solar system (but very, very thin). Surprisingly, given the numbers involved, most of the time genetic replication goes right and embryos are properly formed. However, things can go wrong: At the individual gene level, cystic fibrosis, and at multiple-gene levels, Alzheimer's disease, due to a combination of gene mutation and environmental factors (some breast cancers), and because of damage to chromosomes or chromosomal abnormality (such as a missing chromosome that causes Down's syndrome).

A significant development in reproductive genetics was the discovery of the potency of stem cells and the promise in their medical application. Discovered in mice in 1981, stem cells were isolated in humans in the US in 1998. Basically, animals have two types of cells: somatic and sex or germ line cells. Humans have 220 types of somatic cells that specialize in producing blood, bones, connective tissue, the organs and so on. Sex cells create gametes, sperms and eggs, which are distinguished by their ability to combine with each other to create embryos or to reproduce entire beings. Stem cells have various degrees of power or potency (depending on where they are extracted and at what point in an animal's development) and can divide to form diverse cells types; they are not already specialized like somatic cells. Pluripotent stem cells, found in the inner cell mass (ICM) of five-day-old embryos, can create any kind of cell, somatic or sex cell, but their pluripotency is lost quickly and cannot be found in foetuses, children or adults. ICM pluripotent cells can be developed in the lab and are known as embryonic stem cells. In 2007, scientists managed to reprogramme human adult somatic cells to return to being pluripotent stem cells. Stem cell research and development holds out great promise in medical applications, and in 2010 a spinal cord injury was treated with stem cells in the hope of rebuilding the injured area at the cellular genetic level. In 2012, the treatment showed promise in easing some forms of blindness. In 2014, stem cells created insulin-producing cells offering a potential cure for diabetes, and trials began in Japan to treat age-related blind-ness. By 2019, private clinics began to offer both stem cell therapies for a host of illnesses and injuries, and "regenerative medicine" for age-related issues. All such offers come carefully packaged with the word "promise." From a reproductive theory point of view, stem cell lines offer researchers a whole new lab material with which to explore cellular reproduction and animal development and repair.

IVF provided not only the ability to research human genomes at the earliest stage of development, but also the promise of controlling for and correcting genetic abnormalities, damage and disease before days-old embryos the size of a pin head were implanted. It also made available days-old embryos and their very powerful cells. The main implication for reproductive theory here is that we are no longer concerned only with how reproduction works even if the focus has substantially extended from glands and their neural-hormone triggers to the microbiological level, including the relatively new terrain of genes. We now un-derstand reproduction chiefly as powered by cellular genetic replication.

Conclusions

As humans, we have venerated the female form as the continuation of life, and not only human life, longer than we have attempted to explain human reproduction as a biological exchange between men and women. But since we started recording and writing down these explanations, a significant shift occurred, elevating the male contribution to reproduction to near-divine significance. Despite attempts from ancient Greece to the European Renaissance to empirically solve the mystery of human reproduction, a male-dominant explanation for human procreation per-sisted for almost 2,000 years. Practices in human anatomy alongside improvements in visual technologies, especially the microscope in the 1600s, brought theories of human reproduction closer to how we understand it today, first in terms of reproductive components: the testes, the ovaries, the sperm and then finally the egg. Then relatively quickly and over about 300 years, came the discovery of the systems essential to the working of these parts including nutrition and communica-tion (blood, then cells), activation (nerves, then hormones), and inheritance (genes).

Although we now understand human reproduction to be the equitable ex-change of genetics from both biological parents, remnants of a theory of a supe-rior male status in reproduction remain. Throughout the development of early and modern theories of reproduction, the main organized religions of the time featured a masculine divinity as the font of all creation, often in human form or represented by a man as an envoy between the divine and the earthly worlds. These belief systems sat at the core of social life (and to some extent still do) and heavily influenced the management of human reproduction on the basis of a divine entity that is both the origin (sacred seed) of human being and being responsible for its afterlife. The early scientific striving to explain the mundane aspects of earth-bound human reproductivity in context of these powerful belief systems did not escape their influence.

Currently, reproductive theory has developed to the point that all female reproductive hormones can be suspended and added back artificially in order to time ovulation precisely for IVF. Human ovaries can be hyperovulated to maximize chances in IVF procedures. In the quest for abilities to transfer and store human gametes and cellular embryos, more has been learned about sex cells and their freezing and nutrition outside of the body. The availability of entire human genetic codes for research at the earliest stage of development has allowed for many developments in human genetics and embryonic development and continues to hold out great promise in medical and pharmaceutical applications. Stem cell lines can now be used to create gametes that can reproduce. None of this is possible without both male and female contributions of their respective reproductive matter and the socio-politics of reproduction; the question remains as to how we value such. Medical students are still taught about the "massive and passive egg" and the "brave and motile sperm." Also important is the background pressure from financial interests on theoretical development that is quickly spun into lucrative applications in both genetics and new reproductive technologies.

Further reading

Aristotle, and A. L. Peck. 1943. *Generation of Animals*. Cambridge, MA: Harvard University Press.

Clarke, Adele E. 1998. *Disciplining Reproduction : Modernity, American Life Sciences, and "the Problems of Sex."* Berkeley: University of California Press.

Cobb, Matthew. 2012. "An Amazing 10 Years: The Discovery of Egg and Sperm in the 17th Century." *Reproduction in Domestic Animals* 47 (4): 2–6. DOI: 10.1111/j.1439–0531.2012.02105.x.

Eisler, Riane. 1987. *The Chalice and the Blade—Our History, Our Future*. New York: Harper & Row.

Franklin, Sarah. 2000. "Life Itself: Global Nature and the Genetic Imaginary." In *Global Nature, Global Culture*, edited by Sarah Franklin, Celia Lury, and Jackie Stacey, 256. London: SAGE.

Fujimura, Joan H. 2006. "Sex Genes: A Critical Sociomaterial Approach to the Politics and Molecular Genetics of Sex Determination." *Signs: Journal of Women in Culture and Society* 32 (1): 49–82. DOI: 10.1086/505612.

Gimbutas, Marija. 1989. *The Language of the Goddess*. New York: Harper and Row.

Jacques, Rogers, and Pearce L. Willims. 1997. *Buffon : A Life in Natural History*. Ithaca, NY: Cornell University Press.

Johnson, Martin H. 2011. "Robert Edwards: The Path to IVF." *Reproductive Biomedicine Online* 23: 245–262. DOI: 10.1016%2Fj.rbmo.2011.04.010.

Lesure, Richard. 2002. "The Goddess Diffracted: Thinking About the Figurines of Early Villages." *Current Anthropology* 43 (4): 587–610. DOI: 10.1016/j.rbmo.2011.04.010.

Oudshoorn, Nelly. 1990. "On the Making of Sex Hormones: Research Materials and the Production of Knowledge." *Social Studies of Science* 20 (1): 5–33. DOI: 10.1177/030631290020001001.

Pinto-Correia, Clara. 1997. *The Ovary of Eve: Egg and Sperm and Preformation*. Chicago, IL: University of Chicago Press.

Roberts, Celia. 2008. "Fluid Ecologies—Changing Hormonal Systems of Embodied Difference." In *Bits of Life*, edited by Anneke Smelik and Nina Lykke, 45–60. Seattle and London: University of Washington Press.

Sengoopta, Chandak. 2006. *The Most Secret Quintessence of Life: Sex Glands, and Hormones, 1850–1950*. Chicago, IL: University of Chicago Press.

Shelley, Mary, and Charles. E. Robinson. 2008. *Frankenstein or, The Modern Prometheus*. Oxford: Bodleian Library.

Tuana, Nancy. 1988. "The Weaker Seed and the Sexist Bias of Reproductive Theory." *Hypatia* 3 (1): 35–59. DOI: 10.1111/j.1527–2001.1988.tb00055.x.

Vega, Leslie, and Bret White. 2020. *The Fundamentals of Genetics*. Waltham Abbey, Essex: Ed-Tech Press.

2

THE MEDICALIZATION OF PREGNANCY AND BIRTH

As first natural philosophers, then modern scientists and medical practitioners wrangled over the meaning and function of generation, human reproduction continued without hesitation. Typically, women were attended by other women in their pregnancy and during birth, and in the months following. The attending women were usually known as midwives who passed on their knowledge and experience to other women. Midwives were equipped with knowledge of herbal remedies, techniques for assisting in childbirth, such as turning the foetus *in utero*, and most of all they were equipped with knowledge and experience – handed down over centuries – in managing the human body. Midwives also attended most people in their communities during illness and near death. How then could we reach the point at the start of the 21st century with 98% of US-based births occurring in hospital under the authority of a physician? How is it that pregnancy and birth have become significant parts of medical practice and are treated more as a medical concern than a routine part of human life? How is it that women as midwives were almost completely replaced by a male-dominant medical profession by the start of the 20th century? And, does any of this matter? Below we will examine the process of the modern medicalization of pregnancy and birth as well as resistance to such. We will see how midwives were treated by the emerging profession of modern medicine. We conclude with an assessment of where things stand today in terms of common social practices surrounding human reproduction.

The meaning of medicalization

In the glossy and dense medical textbook, *Clinical Protocols in Obstetrics and Gynecology,* by the clinical professor and physician John Turrentine, we get a good sense of what the current state of medical interventions is in pregnancy and birth.

DOI: 10.4324/9780429467646-3

This text, now in its third edition, is designed to prepare American medical students to write their board exams in the medical specialty unique to females, which focuses on reproductive capacity and health (gynaecology), and pregnancy and birth (obstetrics). There are 410 pages of medical conditions and protocols associated with women's reproductivity, "Obstetrics and gynecology A–Z," starting with abdominal pregnancy (a potentially life-threatening condition that occurs in one out of 7,000 pregnancies) and ending with the drug Zidovudine (used to stop preterm labour). It is a daunting list that includes, for example, 20 different drug protocols used during labour for pain relief, sedation, heartburn, diabetes, hypertension, induction of labour and opening or dilating the cervix. After this extensive list is a concluding section to the text, "Know these for the boards or stay at home," which is useful for finding out what is considered essential to the practice of the specialty. Here we find, for example, the "cardinal movements of labour," which render birth as seven fundamental (almost sacred) movements of the foetus from "engagement" (with the top of the woman's pelvis) to "expulsion" (from the woman's body). These movements of labour match the mechanical metaphor used widely by science to explain reproduction since the 1800s and reflect broader tendencies to reduce and tailor physiologies and functions to satisfy broader interests.

As scientific and medical research and clinical development in reproduction expanded in the 20th century to include cellular biology, biochemistry, endocrinology (hormones) and neurology, pregnancy and birth were increasingly medicalized. Many dysfunctions, illness and disease associated with the reproducing body were identified, opening up opportunities for medical intervention. Almost all of these were in the female reproducing body. Andrology (the male equivalent of gynaecology) as a medical specialty was virtually non-existent during the 20th century. To understand the extent of medicalization of female reproductivity we need to turn to the margins of "home" or "natural" birth movements; we also need to understand the process of medicalization and its critics.

The medical textbook on contemporary OB/GYN protocols stands as a prime example of how pregnancy and birth are now deemed worthy of considerable medical attention. Of course, reproduction or the generation of humans has long occurred, and certainly well before the establishment of modern healthcare, a fact which has engaged sociologists, philosophers and historians and led to the development of critical theories of medicalization. But first, Elliane Riska in her analysis of gender and the medicalization thesis notes how the American sociologist Talcott Parsons coined the term "medical sociology" to flag the centrality of medicine to modern social life. Known as someone who viewed the good society as a well-oiled, stable and predictable machine of distinct but interactive parts or social institutions – such as schools, governing bodies – and normal behaviours or norms, Parsons viewed the rising influence of medicine in the social world as benign and helpful, and an example of how modern societies were more civic and less dogmatic than those that came before. Medicine, not religious authorities, now regulated social deviance, and an individual was not held morally responsible for a diagnosable illness, such as hyperactivity; you were not a bad boy but had a medical condition. From this perspective, which dominated social studies of medicine from the mid-20th century to the 1970s, clear and consistent medical professional roles, a specific division of labour, and formal education were parts of the necessary social system for managing health and keeping the social world stable. So the medicalization of pregnancy and birth was, and largely is still, considered a good and necessary thing to properly manage the risky business of reproduction, which, in turn, is central to the future of society.

Throughout the 1970s, views on medicalization became more critical. Initially the critique involved the monopolization of medical knowledge, as by the American sociologist Eliot Freidson, who argued that medical knowledge was kept secret by medical authorities to protect their professional autonomy. This helps explain how the road to the current dominance of physicians in healthcare involved wresting authority from long-serving professions, including midwives. The sociologist Irving Zola added that the medical system had moved beyond the mandate of keeping societies healthy and stable to practising a form of social control. Rather than this being a conscious programme of the medical profession, Zola and others saw this shift as a result of the increased medicalization of daily life. This medicalized sociality is based on an implicit social contract between patients, healthcare providers and "the medical industrial complex" (identified by American physician and social commentator Stanley Wohl). Medicalization was presented as necessary to handle increasingly risky life, and egged on by commercial interests, the medical industrial complex, which continued to unveil threats to human health. One of the impacts of this medicalization thesis raised by Zola's student, Peter Conrad, was that nonmedical issues became defined and treated as such. "Treating" pregnancy and birth – even providing these normal human functions with their own medical specialty – is a prime example of and was at the core of feminist medicalization theories that emerged in the late 1970s building on these initial criticisms of medicalization.

The list of protocols in Turrentine's contemporary medical textbook includes "manoeuvres" (the nine methods used to move the foetus into proper position for birth) and almost all of these manoeuvres are named after the medical men recognized as the creators of the techniques. Besides generating a rationale for largely male and exclusive physician authority over pregnancy and birth, this modern example of medical reproductive practice effectively erases centuries of midwifery practice that included moving the foetus *in utero* just prior to birth, as well as performing caesarean sections (C-sections) as early as the 1400s in France. The appropriation and elimination of roles long served by predominantly female midwives, followed by the medicalization of female reproduction, drew criticism starting in the late 1970s from feminist sociologists of medicine as well as from largely white, North American middle-class activists calling for home or natural birth. In Europe, as with economically strapped regions throughout the world, midwifery continued as a profession, although rarely as independent of the medicalization of pregnancy and birth.

The American sociologist long concerned with women and reproduction, Barbara Katz Rothman, noted how the medicalization of birth did not go unchallenged, even by members of the early medical profession. Initially European doctors Dick Grantly-Reed (England) and Ferdinand Lamaze (France) gained enormous attention and a strong following by pregnant and birthing women for their efforts to pull back on the extent of American-based medicalization reached by the mid-20th century. The American practices included completely anaesthetizing labouring women, shaving their pubic hair before birth and routinely cutting the vaginal opening (episiotomy) during birth. More importantly, the American approach relied on the birthing woman as a passive and compliant participant in birth and created a dependency on medical authorities to make it through the process safely: doctors, not mothers, delivered babies. On a related matter, this was also the time of the mass marketing of formula feeding babies with stamps of approval from medical authorities. Some women and women's groups spoke out against and organized alternatives to these trends, but rather than it being a revolution, Katz Rothman describes this resistance as a "reformation." These calls to "natural" and "home" births worked within rather than against the medical model. Typical of this time of quasi-activism is the list of instructions prepared by pregnant women for their obstetricians, indicating the opted-out procedures such as routine episiotomy and pubic shaving and the level of pain relief the women wanted during labour. These requests were often derided by physicians who, by this time, had the legal authority and responsibility to act in the best interests of their patients according to the protocols of medical training, which heavily medicalized pregnancy and birth: The doctor knows best. This public criticism of medicalized birth is actually reflected in the 2008 Turrentine medical textbook as: "Routine episiotomy is no longer indicated and should be used only in selective cases." The return of a restricted midwifery practice in various states and provinces throughout North America is also a result of this resistance to medicalization trends.

Within the litigious and private medical healthcare delivery system in the US, Yvonne Brackbill (PhD), June Rice (a lawyer) and Diony Young (a childbirth educator) wrote a guide in the mid-1980s for "consumer groups" of obstetric healthcare to navigate the legalities of high-tech obstetrics and to use them to take some control over their maternity care. This tactic points to how increased medical attention and technological intervention in pregnancy and birth, especially in a private healthcare context, resulted in higher rates of litigation when the risky business of birth went wrong. American obstetricians pay among the highest annual rates for malpractice insurance: in 2020 about $85,000–$200,000. Indeed, Gena Corea, a US-based feminist commentator on reproductive health, published the book, *The Hidden Malpractice*, a decade earlier detailing examples of largely unabated medical experimentation on women in the name of scientific and healthcare advances, especially as almost all American women enter the medical system at some time in their life because of their reproductive capacity. The prevailing gender norms resulted in an obstetric-gynaecological specialty whose authority figures were chiefly men, and whose patients, who were all people needing obstetric care, were not expected to question authority. Brackbill and her colleagues' guide was designed to help birthing women use this situation to their advantage by evoking legal authority.

The level of experimentation and malpractice in women's reproductive health is evident in the thalidomide disaster. In the 1950s, the West German pharmaceutical company, Chemie Grunenthal GmbH, developed the drug thalidomide initially as an anti-convulsive drug, but which was also found to be effective in treating morning sickness during pregnancy. Although the drug was tested for overdose (none found), it was never tested for effects on pregnant women or developing foetuses. It was first released prescription-free (or over the counter) in Germany and much of Europe in 1956, and by prescription in the UK and Japan in 1958, followed by Norway in 1959, and Australia in 1960. By 1960, doctors became concerned about its side effects: patients using the drug long term reported numbness and tingling in their hands and feet, and by 1961 a link between the drug use in pregnant women and children born with missing or malformed limbs, hands and feet was made independently by two doctors, one Australian and one German. In the end, 10,000 children were born worldwide with thalidomide-caused deformations. The drug was withdrawn from the UK and Germany at the end of 1961, with all other countries following suit soon after. It was never approved for use in the US thanks to the persistence of a Canadian doctor Frances Kelsey, working for the US Food and Drug Agency at the time, who insisted that the pharmaceutical distributor demonstrate that it was safe for pregnant women; it did not. Ironically, Canada did approve and distribute the drug for several months in 1961 and as a result more than 100 people living in Canada were born with thalidomide-related disabilities.

Other experiments involving pregnant women include diaethylstilbestrol (DES – a synthetic oestrogen hormone) used between 1938 and 1971 in millions of women to help prevent miscarriage. DES was eventually found to cause increased rates of breast cancer, other reproductive cancers and infertility in the children of these women. Both of these cases led to more stringent measures for testing drugs with particular attention to pregnant and nursing women, but only after widespread and tragic consequences.

Concerns for the overmedicalization of pregnancy and birth persist, with a current focus on rates of C-section births. According to a 2018 study appearing in the highly ranked medical journal, *The Lancet,* most developed countries have a C-section rate of 25%, with the US, China and Australia at about 30%, and the Dominican Republic, Turkey, Egypt and Brazil with rates above 50%. The global rate has almost doubled since 2000, and many birth activists and physicians are calling for a reduction in unnecessary use of this major surgical intervention in women giving birth. There are also concerns for the foetus born via C-section over lost benefits from vaginal birth (chiefly respiratory and immune system development). By contrast, in developing countries, criticisms of medicalization usually arise in terms of missing or inadequate healthcare infrastructure rather than unnecessary medical intervention experienced at the individual patient level.

Concern for the medicalization of daily life continues but has altered significantly in its approach. Biomedicalization is the term used today to define a multi-focal analysis of what is going on in medicine, which according to the American sociologist of health, Adele Clark and others, includes the interaction of biomedical knowledge, technologies, services and capital. The addition of "bio" to medical knowledge recognizes developments particularly in genetics, and the tight interactions between medicine and genetic science. This gives rise to biomedical health (not only illness, injury and disease), and to the ever more sophisticated delivery of high-tech healthcare in the name of prevention and health enhancement. Finally, biomedicine is seen to effect people in new ways, not only as individual bodies but as populations or groups of bodies, both with significant consequences for social identities. This recognition that medicalization is different and experienced differently among various populations according to social and political contexts helps explain the seeming contradiction between perceived over medicalization of birth in developed countries and under medicalization in sub-developed countries. Many people in sub- or undeveloped nations cannot access necessary basic healthcare for the health problems stemming from poverty that particularly affect reproducing women and young children, such as poor nutrition and heavy-water carrying, leading to malformed and small pelvises that complicate birth, and unsafe drinking water which results in deadly water-borne diseases especially in newborns and young children.

Midwifery: professionalization and medicalization

The American social critic and activist Barbara Ehrenreich, with academic and former editor of the progressive American magazine, *Mother Jones*, Deidre English, documented how women were historically removed from positions of traditional authority over healing and birth, starting with the European witch-hunts in 16th century continental Europe and spreading to England and Scotland shortly afterwards. Numbers of chiefly women (estimated at 85% of those persecuted as witches) who were put to cruel deaths vary from the hundreds of thousands to several million over about 200 years. Various women-denigrating rationales came into play to send women to their deaths, including the Original Sin of Eve, the demonization of female sexual desire and the blaming of women for upsetting natural balances. Women, especially those with any social influence, were blamed for crop failures, disease, male impotence and "monstrous" births. Many of these women derived their perceived power (and threat) from the traditional and informal authority vested in them over centuries as midwives and healers. Even though throughout the witch-hunt there were male physicians, including the first gynaecologists, they rarely practised their art on actual patients, and they were protected by their gender. It was typically a woman's job to attend to the pregnant, the ill and the dying. With the developments in science, its increasing authority over knowledge and the development of modern medicine as practice, midwives and traditional healers became problematic and symbolic of cruder and uneducated times, and the well-being of the human body and mind became a highly contested ground.

There is a substantial amount written about midwifery historically, and how contemporary midwifery practices compare with the medical model of pregnancy and birth. Because of the significant impact of medicalization generally, current midwifery practices are not the same as they were. Nor is there a single form of midwifery practised over the centuries and in the same way today around the world. There are, however, commonalities in how modern medicine and its typical male medical practitioner replaced women midwives and took authority over what had long been their domain as healers and attendants of pregnant and birthing women.

The British historian Jean Donnison provides an overview of midwifery from early history – the midwives, Shirpak and Puah, appear in the *Torah* and the Bible written about 400 BCE – to the late 20th century as midwifery was either rejected by or assumed into the medical model and made to report to medical authorities. Before this, childbearing was long considered women's business, as depicted in the 2nd-century CE (Common Era) bas-relief or sculpted plaque on the tomb of the Roman midwife Scribonia Attica, which shows two women attending a third woman during childbirth: one attendant holds the labouring woman upright on a stool, as the midwife kneels before her with her hand between the birthing woman's legs, examining her. Although we have spotty details about midwifery practice from early history through medieval Europe and beyond, it is believed that a respected midwife required experience of childbirth herself, and the more experience, the better. Also, a mature woman, who had experience with the healing arts (usually a combination of rituals and herb-based remedies), was favoured. This preference helps explain why midwives were caught up as victims in the witch-hunt, as these older women had the respect of their communities for what they knew (neither for their sexual allure nor for their reproductive capacity) and attended moments of life and death as an authority figure. They were also early businesswomen who often supported themselves with their practice. In an era that ordained masculine privilege, these women were out of bounds, and their inquisitors sought to put them back in their proper place.

The professionalization of modern healthcare was predominantly controlled and peopled by male physicians, and modern medical practice threatened to eliminate midwifery as a competitor for business and authority. However, midwifery was practised almost continuously alongside physicians from the earliest known doctors in classical Greece and with the early (barber and barbarous) surgeons of the Middle Ages. Physicians, including obstetricians, gynaecologists and surgeons, numbered a few women among them from time to time, such as the celebrated Greek surgeon, gynaecologist and obstetrician, Aspasia (about 300 CE), and Cecelia of Oxford who was hired in the mid-14th century as court surgeon by Queen Philippa (wife of Edward III of England). And while the fathers of classic medicine, including Aristotle who was among the first to explain the generation of humans, relied on midwives for information, especially practical experience of pregnancy and birth, women were typically denied access to education that would allow them participation in medicine throughout the ages in any meaningful number. Globally, many universities at the turn of the 20th century forbade or severely restricted women's access to modern medical schools. In 2017, the Association of American Medical Colleges announced that for the first time in its history the number of women enrolled in US medical schools was slightly more (50.7%) than that of men. According to the 2018 report of Universities UK, the rate here is slightly higher at about 58% female enrollment, but these figures include dentistry as well as medicine. A key explanation for these developments is the extension of public education to girls as well as boys, and the emancipation of women in the public sphere of work.

According to Ehrenreich and English, the established medical profession of the 19th century turned to "cleaning up" the problem of midwifery (and other traditional healing arts) by denouncing it as a sound practice in the face of all that science was now unearthing, with only appropriately trained professionals capable of handling the complex world of human health, including pregnancy and birth. Richard and Dorothy Wertz examined how hospitalized birth became the norm in 1920s America as the "fashion changed" and traditional midwifery associated with very old rituals and even magic gave way to safer scientific methods of modern medicine. Less than 5% of women in the US delivered their babies in hospitals at the turn of the 20th century; today less than 2% of US births occur outside of hospitals. Even in countries such as The Netherlands, where midwifery never disappeared and functions today independent of oversight by physicians, home birth is limited to about 30%.

The regulation of midwifery occurred over two major periods: during the 14th and 15th centuries with the move from religious authority to civic governance, and then again around the turn of the 20th century when medical professions were legally recognized and their respective scopes were defined. Midwifery came under formal control of emerging governments in Europe as early as the 14th century, partly as a reaction to the drummed-up social fear of the magic or "witchcraft" (typically incantations and the application of herbal remedies) that midwives used while attending women. In the infamous document, *The Hammer of Witches* (1486), the German inquisitors Springer and Institorus claim that midwives "surpass all other witches in their crimes." During the Inquisition, women were accused of and executed for the murdering of babies at birth and for killing foetuses in the womb as signs of their compact with the Devil. "Monstrous births" (anomalies in foetuses, newborns and stillborn foetuses) were often first witnessed by midwives, and during the religious fervour that gave rise to the witch-hunt, they or the mother were often held morally responsible. As democracies formed, municipal-level governments were struck with health responsibilities, thanks partly to the Plague when bodies and infections had to be managed in densely populated cities and towns (despite any knowledge of sterile technique and little known about microbiological conta-gion). Midwifery was included as a health concern: the first formal act to control midwifery in England came in 1512. About half a century before, there were similar moves in Germany and France. Unlike the religious-sanctioned witch-hunt, these civic regulations were more concerned with the scope of practice al-lowed to the midwife rather than with the midwives' moral character. Donnison points out how by regulating midwifery in terms of ability and scope or practice, the mainly female midwife profession was distinguished from a growing body of medical men now interested in birth, and women were effectively barred from their traditional body of knowledge, practices and technologies. An important but not the sole example of how this shift took place is found in the case of the Chamberlen family.

Donnison describes how between the late 1500s and the 1880s, almost the entire male membership of the British Chamberlen family tried to insert them-selves into the rising and potentially lucrative business of delivery practice by physicians. In order to make a decent living at assisting women during child-birth, the Chamberlens focused their attention on the wealthy and the influ-ential and sold their services as keeping up moral standards of decency during birth, which they achieved through a growing custom to drape the birthing woman. In 1647, Peter Chamberlen published *Voice in Rhama, or, the Crie of Women and Children*, arguing against traditional midwifery as something lowly, and of the uneducated and unrefined. However, this family of birth practi-tioners (but not physicians) was forced to become licensed as midwives, and they never fully won over birthing women's trust from traditional midwives. The family persisted, nonetheless, and further distinguished itself in its male midwifery-like practice with a secret device. A visit to most museums of mod-ern healthcare usually includes a display of the barbaric instruments used in early surgery in general, and in particular the devices used to compact and extract blocked foetuses during birth. What the Chamberlens offered was a device purported to ease troubled deliveries and to save the mother and perhaps even the child in the process. Using a scissor-like, spooned tool (what we now call forceps), the Chamberlens would attempt to deliver women, especially the wealthy and royalty, in a way unmatched in traditional midwifery and even in obstetrics. They enjoyed substantial financial success, which was secured for over 200 years by keeping the technique and tool from view: the modesty drapes no doubt helping, along with a special locked storage box. This tactic to keep knowledge and tools away from traditional birth attendants was repeated soon after by the emerging profession of medical practitioners that helped effect a transfer of authority from traditional midwives to physicians specializing in women's reproductive health and birth.

Contemporary arguments used against the practice of midwifery grew out of indicators of social progress defined by the Industrial Revolution. Thanks to the development of statistical sciences and bureaucratic methods, rates of health and well-being of populations were collected and tracked. The rates of death of mothers at birth (maternal mortality) and the death of infants at or immediately following birth (infant mortality) became key players in the near-elimination and medicalization of midwifery in the modern period. Up until the first quarter of the 20th century, the great majority of births throughout pre-modern Europe, colonial North America, Australia and New Zealand took place at home under the care of a midwife or wise woman, who may or may not have been licensed by earlier regulations; there were very few "lying-in" hospitals used for delivery until this point. And mortality rates became significant: The sociologist Cecelia Benoit notes how infant mortality in Sweden during the 1920s, for example, was recorded at about 60 deaths per 1,000 (today's rate for Sweden is 2.3 per 1,000). Although these initial high mortality rates owed more to the lack of knowledge in germ theory and sterile practice along with risky surgical interventions in difficult births than to midwifery practice, these rates became powerful weapons in rationalizing the medicalization of pregnancy and birth and in removing midwives from the scene.

Infant and maternal mortality rates were only kept reliably once medical practice started to take hold; hospitalization and medicalization of birth, including medically sanctioned midwifery, were included in this data collection. The lack of any prior data makes it impossible to compare risk and outcomes between traditional midwifery and early medical obstetrics. However, even these early attempts to track the cause of infant and maternal mortality rates were tricky to read, especially by profession. Some midwives were medically trained, while some were not; some were trained effectively, while some were not; some labours started with a contracted midwife, but were then transferred to a physician because of complications; sometimes such transfers were fully documented, while sometimes they were not; some attending physicians were obstetrically trained, while some were not. But this did not stop many early medical associations and physicians from accusing traditional midwives of inferior healthcare and worse, and from arguing that childbirth should fall under the authority of physicians to improve outcomes for the mother and the child.

The physician and medical historian Irvine Loudon claims that if you asked an American obstetrician in the early 20th century what they thought of midwives,

> you would have been told that the midwife was typically old, ignorant and filthy, 'not far removed from the jungles of Africa, gin-fingering, guzzling… with her brains full of snuff, her fingers full of dirt and her brains full of arrogance and superstition'.

Besides employing the force of socially-accepted sexism and racism to demean midwives, physicians also downplayed their own interests in the professional monopolization of education, techniques and tools; the harmful effects of medical experimentation; the exposure of hospitalized patients to contagious disease; and how poverty and poor nutrition significantly increased risks to women and children in or near childbirth.

After carefully combing through American and UK statistics in this period on maternal mortality rates by who attended the birth, the mother's class and race, Loudon unearths significant contradictions in the medical profession's claims that midwifery provided an inferior quality of maternity care. One contradiction is found in the "reverse social class connection," which is a higher rate of maternal mortality among the middle classes than the lower classes in London, UK; as expected, infant mortality rates were higher in the city's slums, due to very poor living conditions, untreated disease and malnutrition. But why would middle-class women giving birth be dying at a higher rate than slum-dwelling, lower-class mothers? In a 1930–1932 study of England and Wales' maternal mortality rates according to class, rates of maternal death were the lowest among the lowest-class women compared to all women studied for all categories: 3.32 of the lowest class of women dying per 1,000 while giving birth compared to 3.70 of all other, higher classes of birthing women. This unexpected discrepancy was due to the risk of contagious disease (puerperal fever) and illness ripping through maternity wards in hospitals. Midwife-assisted birth in the home was not exposed to this disease.

In the US, which around the same time had the highest maternal mortality rate in the Western world, risky birth was complicated by race and the pernicious combination of racialization and poverty. The highest rates of maternal mortality were found in the South within rural, extremely poor Black communities, where Black midwives were the primary birth attendants. Black birthing women in South Carolina between 1934 and 1935 died at the rate of 215 women per 1,000 births compared to 128 for their white neighbours, who were normally attended to by physicians at birth. The culprit here was poor training of midwives, especially in antiseptic practices, to control puerperal fever and infection. Once properly trained, notes Loudon, these same midwives brought the maternal mortality rate below that of areas where physician–attended birth was common.

A 1926 US Department of Labour comparison of 1920s maternal mortality rates by the usual attendant (midwife, doctor or a combination of the two) between north western European countries, the US, Australia and New Zealand reveals Denmark with the lowest rate (23.5 deaths per 10,000 births) where only midwives usually attend birth, and the US with the highest rate (79.9) where doctors predominantly attend birth. The rates are tightly associated with the type of attendant: where only midwives typically attend the rates are under 30; where doctors predominantly attend the rates are over 60. Where both may attend, the rate falls between 30 and 60. Despite the characterization of midwives by members of the emerging medical profession as inept, crazed and a risk to reproducing women, it was initially far more risky for women to have their children in hospital under the care of physicians than having their child at home with a midwife.

The effectiveness of midwifery, along with a growing medical practice to triage pregnancies by potential risk, may be the reason why in most countries where universal healthcare and a welfare state were established by the mid-20th century, midwifery was granted a substantial place within or beside medical obstetrics. In

Sweden by the 1930s, maternity care was publicly funded, midwife-focused and in a tiered medical model from midwifery-based centres to physician-focused care and hospitalization for high-risk cases. In the Netherlands, maternal care was independently operated by freelance midwives, who have been recognized legally as independent caregivers since 1865. Later, maternal care was included in the medical system for high-risk cases. In the UK, it was a combination of the two approaches from the start of modern medical practice with midwifery professionally recognized in 1902 and divided between hospital-based midwives and community-based midwives with hospital-admitting privileges. In the US, where there is no universal healthcare and thus no provision for effective maternal care for all, and where medicine, especially obstetrics, is big business with powerful medical lobbies, the recognition of midwifery has always been spotty and usually allowed only in places where medicine did not want to venture (poor rural areas for example, out of fear by doctors of not being paid). Later, US midwives aligned with the nursing profession to have the practice of nurse-midwives legally recognized in 1955, but by far the majority of births today are attended by obstetricians in hospitals (about 95%). Australia, as with most British colonies, imported midwifery with its settlers and legally recognized it in 1915; but like Canada, midwife-attended home births were largely replaced starting in the early 20th century by hospital ones, overseen by physicians who assumed the role of typical birth attendant. Canada was last among the Western countries to legally recognize midwifery starting in 1994. Here, middle-class, white women adopted the critical medicalization perspective (pregnancy and birth are unproblematic and low risk most of the time and do not require automatic and extensive medical attention) and lobbied for a de-medicalization of pregnancy and birth as provincial governments recognized the potential for significant savings in public healthcare (midwives and birthing centres cost far less than obstetricians and hospital beds).

Racialized geopolitics of reproductive health and childbirth

The battle for authority over women's reproducing bodies is complicated by racialization and geopolitics. Medicalization alongside social stratification fills out the picture, and the US provides a brutal example. The historian Marie Schwartz explains how between 1808 – when the US stopped the import of slaves – and 1863 – when President Abraham Lincoln issued the Emancipation Proclamation freeing all enslaved people in the US – the interests of slave owners and physicians combined and they jointly turned their attention to slave women's reproductivity. Despite the end of the slave trade, anyone born into slavery in the US before its abolition was considered a slave, so "birthing a slave" was an important and urgent business. To directly maintain the fortunes of plantation owners in the South and the political economy of the entire nation (especially the Northeast), enslaved Black women's reproduction became a precious commodity. All available resources were brought to bear, including physicians overseeing slave women's reproductive health, starting when they reached adolescence and continuing throughout their childbearing years, all at the slave owners' cost. This investment in human capital was also used to dispel rising criticisms of slavery by pointing to how well slave owners cared for their slaves. The near half-century opportunity of physicians' access to Black women's bodies, against their will, played a central role in the medicalization of pregnancy and birth, and to the development of gynaecology in and beyond the US.

As with women elsewhere, Afro-American women had a strong cultural history of community-based, lay women's attendance during pregnancy and birth, and one which continued after emancipation and well into the 20th century. Indeed, when slave owners brought doctors in to ensure the future and well-being of their slave stock, the physicians often met with resistance and noncompliance. However, these women were slaves and their choices were severely and violently limited. This brings us to the Alabama-based doctor J. Marion Simms, considered the "father" of modern gynaecology, who served as president of both the American Medical Association and the American Gynecological Association. Simms surgically experimented, without anaesthetic, on slave women around the mid-19th century to address a complication of birth that impeded future reproduction. According to the 1850 census, Simms owned 17 slaves, of which 12 were female. Some were patients and some were assistants to his experiments. It is possible some women were bought for the express purpose of experimentation. Simms was investigating a surgical solution to what was then considered medically to be one of the most significant obstacles to successful reproduction: reproductive fistulae.

As with reproductive theory, 18th-century medical science in general focused on the body as a mechanism, and so it was with labour and birth, particularly in terms of obstruction of the birthing foetus. The Chamberlen's forceps were their response to this problem, and by the 18th century, these were finally well known and widely in use by physicians. Other tools to help remove an obstructed foetus included those designed to perform craniotomies on the foetus *in utero*. All of these instruments typically had very poor outcomes, especially at the onset of their use. The birthing foetus commonly perished, and often so did the mother due to perforations, haemorrhage and infection. The cause of obstructed birth was understood as one of size: the pelvis was considered too small and/or the birthing foetus' head was too large. Using European women's pelvic size and shape as a norm, many women of African origin were found to have smaller and more shallow pelvises and thus Afro-American slaves were deemed more prone to obstructed labour. There is some congenital cause to the formation of bone structures, and there are today high rates of complications due to obstructed birth and prolonged labour, concentrated in some African countries. However, virtually no attention was paid in 19th-century southeastern US states to early adolescent pregnancy, chronic malnutrition and heavy work among slaves that can result in small and misshapen pelvises and may lead to difficult and damaging births. Today obstructed birth and prolonged labour among chronically malnourished women and in very young women who must carry heavy weights (such as water) early on in their lives are understood as tightly interconnected. Obstructed and prolonged reproductive labour can tear the tissue between the birth canal (the vagina) and the neighbouring bladder (creating a vesico-vaginal fistula) or rectum (creating a recto-vaginal fistula). A fistula is not often fatal but leaves the woman in a state of chronic leaking from the bladder or rectum, which has disastrous social consequences and leaves such women with little social contact and virtually no chances to continue with intimate relationships. In other words, slave women who suffered from reproductive fistulae were often no longer reproducing. Instruments including forceps, catheters and the tools to perform foetal craniotomy, as well as pessaries (made of bone, metal and ivory) placed in the vagina by doctors to keep a prolapsed or extruding uterus in place, if not used or placed properly (which was often the case) could also create fistulae. At the time when Simms was conducting his experiments (mid-19th century) many physicians admitted that most vaginal tearing was caused by inexperienced colleagues using instruments during birth.

It was the surgical technique to repair these tears and to return continence and a profitable reproductive life to women suffering from them that preoccupied the Alabama doctor in his barbaric experiments on slave women. One of these women, Anarcha, underwent 30 surgeries over three and a half years, all without anaesthetic. Her initial fistula appeared right after Simms attended her extended labour and used forceps, with which he was not very experienced. Simms left Alabama in 1852 for a lucrative and illustrious career in New York City, where he applied his now successful surgical technique on white women, who received anaesthesia and were no doubt enormously grateful to be spared the shame and social isolation that reproductive fistulae bring. Some argue, especially physicians, that the successful development of the technique (widely in use today) justifies Simms' means of perfecting it. Without a doubt, the literally captive population of reproducing slave women in the development of medical interventions in female reproductivity sits at an extreme and racially violent end of a continuum of medical attention to pregnancy and birth. This case also demonstrates how broader sets of interests, especially financial ones, figure in their medicalization. It was also an isolated period of medical attention to Afro-Americans, which was followed by over a century of medical inattention and lack of public health resources to the children of slaves in what became a deeply racist and segregated society following their so-called emancipation. Deadly inequitable access to reproductive health and medicine according to race in the US continues today.

By the start of the 20th century in most Western nations, death rates in general, including infant mortality, were on the decline except for maternal mortality, which remained steady. Exposure of women in crowded maternity wings and hospitals to experimental procedures and inexperienced physicians relatively new to the birthing bedside, along with the germs and disease doctors brought with them from other patients, are all likely contributors to the rise in death and infant mortality rates in the early 1900s. What were things like in under-developed nations?

Lenore Manderson, a medical anthropologist, unearths a 1936 report of a British doctor, Mary Blacklock, on the welfare of women and children in the colonies of Hong Kong, Malaya, Ceylon, Palestine, China, Burma and India. Blacklock determines that throughout this expansive area with their large and diverse populations, colonization did not bring to women and children here the benefits of health and education enjoyed at home. Both infant and maternal mortality rates remained high, and applying Western standards of nutrition and cleanliness was unrealistic as many had only rice to eat and had no access to clean, warm water. Precociously in terms of global development, Blacklock pointed to the tight connection between the education of girls and positive health outcomes for their families, including lower reproductive mortality rates.

This example of the exportation of the modern medicalization of pregnancy and birth illuminates the characteristics of modern development practices, namely to attempt to transfer the benefits of a developed country to one less developed. Maternity and infant mortality rates operated and continue to operate as highly significant indicators of development, as they are associated with social levels of nutrition, healthcare and education, which, in turn, are connected to broader socio-economic and political stabilities. This dominant approach often functions at the expense of local traditions, including local healthcare and socio-cultural practices surrounding reproducing women.

In 2006, the World Health Organization (WHO) produced the document: *Reproductive Health Indicators: Guidelines for their Generation, Interpretation, and Analysis for Global Monitoring.* This 63-page document provides the specific statistical methods for determining and standardizing rates associated with reproductive health that are tracked by this global health watchdog. Some of the indicators of what constitutes reproductive health are familiar, such as maternal mortality, perinatal (newborn) mortality and access to skilled professional healthcare. Beyond the confines of medicalization of women's active reproductivity, a globalized definition of reproductive health now takes into account factors such as the general health of women (anaemia, and the presence of sexually transmitted diseases such as syphilis and HIV), socio-medical factors ("contraception prevalence" and "percentage of obstetric and gynaecological admissions owing to abortion") and one male indicator: "incidence of urethritis in men." There are also indicators for levels of education regarding HIV prevention practices and contraceptive use. WHO reports in 2018 that 83 per 10,000 women die from preventable causes related to pregnancy and childbirth (the highest risk among adolescent women under the age of 15), and that 99% of maternal deaths occur in developing countries. WHO's goal is to reduce worldwide maternal mortality to less than 7 per 10,000 births. They recognize the role of medically trained midwives as "essential" to meeting this target, likely due to the inability of these places to afford the Western medicalization of pregnancy and birth featuring physician-based care in a hospital.

Tensions play through this progressive vision for global reproductive health reduced to a list of socio-medical indicators that is culturally and racially problematic. The profound self-identification of peoples around the world includes how they view and live their reproductivity. For example, in a study of contemporary indigenous experiences of pregnancy and birth in Canada, edited by Hannah Tait Neufeld and Jaime Cidro, "the repatriation of birth" and "birth on the land" refer to responses to centuries-long, community-destroying effects of Western colonization. "Residential schools" are an infamous part of an intentional and systematic campaign by Canadian governments and the Catholic Church that ripped apart ties between Indigenous children and their families and communities, their land and the experience of living on it, and which almost eradicated their languages, rituals and way of being in the world. The last residential school in Canada was closed in 1996. In 2021, 215 bodies of Indigenous children were discovered in unmarked graves immediately outside a former residential school in British Columbia.

The impact of this cultural genocide on pregnancy and birth involves intergenerational family breakdown and the loss of support and modelling for new parents, substance abuse, poor nutrition due to intergenerational poverty and the sexual violation and murder of especially young Indigenous women at rates far above national averages. The routine airlifting of women to regional hospitals for pregnancy monitoring and childbirth may provide a stopgap measure to the substandard living conditions forced on these people over centuries, and certainly addresses high-risk pregnancies and births, but it does little to address the socio-culture ruptures in Indigenous peoples' experiences and traditions surrounding pregnancy and birth. The social anthropologist Rachel Olson, who has studied Canadian Indigenous women's birth experiences and the evacuation of Indigenous women from their communities and culture to far away and alien hospitals, addresses biomedical risks, but not socio-cultural risks, and prioritizes the former at the risk of the later.

Almost identical histories spell out for the Maori in New Zealand where Maori maternal knowledges and associated practices are now under a process of reclamation. While in places that sit between development and underdevelopment, such as the areas on either side of the Mexico-US border, matters are more complex, and contradictions of capital abound. For example, Candace Johnson points to how Canadian midwives sought training experience on poor Mexican women as Canada slowly came to legally recognize midwifery in the 1990s. Johnson explains this contradiction in birth experiences as based in material realities: women with economic means have the ability to resist medicalization and insist on a return to so-called natural practices as an individual preference; pregnancy and birth is a private matter and an individual right. For systemically poor women, pregnancy and birth is better understood in terms of intersecting inequalities, such as poverty, the effects of colonization and racialization. In Cuba, the UK and Canada, where the medicalization of pregnancy and birth is well established and in principle available to all equally through universal healthcare, women of means are found to knowingly negotiate higher-quality healthcare and more reproductive choice. All three countries enjoy among the lowest maternal and infant mortality rates in the world.

Conclusions

There are two forces at play in the current state of medicalization of pregnancy and birth. One surrounds the rise of modern medicine over the last century and a half, how it became an authority over pregnancy and birth and how this has been received. The other has to do with the professionalization of medicine and how that relates to a very long tradition of women attending women during pregnancy and birth. Without question our lives are lived far more under the sway of medical authority. We have never been so medically screened, and now have internalized the responsibility for our health through what we eat, how we supplement our diets, how much and how well we sleep, whether we can feel suspicious lumps in our bodies, how often we exercise and to what extent in terms of heart rate, steps taken and so on. Pregnancy and birth were caught early on in this trend of constant monitoring and internalized medical concern. What was long recognized as an intense, risky yet everyday matter, became the focus of considerable medical attention, alongside illness, injury and disease. Drives behind the switch vary, from stated concerns over infant and maternal mortality rates to less obvious interests in medical experimentation and financial profit.

During this significant transfer of authority from women birth attendants to physicians worldwide, contradictions abound. Although early modern medicine claimed it would provide safer outcomes to mothers and babies than what traditional midwifery could offer, the initial movement of women to hospitals increased mortality rates due to exposure to infectious disease, and to interventions by physicians using instruments with which they were poorly trained or untrained to use. Despite fierce opposition to midwifery by the emerging profession of modern gynaecology and obstetrics in some places, notably North America, many other countries combined (and continue to combine) midwifery and medical practice in stepped systems with varying rates of medical authority and medicalization of pregnancy and birth. Although modern medicine was often presented as a benefit to whole populations, and healthy pregnancies and safe deliveries for all citizens remain important indicators of social progress today, healthcare delivery, including that surrounding reproduction, is highly determined by economic means and differs among specific populations within nations and between so-called developed and developing nations. Although modern medicine's prime stated objective is the well-being of individuals, the barbaric history of early medical attention to Afro-American slaves in the 19th century demonstrates how financial interest (involving in this case slave owners, aspiring physicians and the American economy) determines medical practice. Finally, although modern medicine is aligned with contemporary principles of science, the profession of physicians, initially dominated by white men, monopolized medical knowledge on the basis of shaky theories of gendered and racialized intelligence, long preventing many women and others from marginalized populations a place in medical practice, including attending women during pregnancy and birth.

Further reading

Benoit, Cecilia. 1991. *Midwives in Passage: The Modernization of Maternity Care.* St. John's: Institute of Social and Economic Research, Memorial University.

Boerma, Ties, Carine Ronsman, Dessalegn Melesse, Alusisio Barros, Fernando Barros, Liang Juan, and Ann-Beth Moller. 2018. "Global epidemiology of use of and disparities in caesarian sections." *The Lancet*, June 23, 2021, 1341–1348, October 13, 2018. https://www.thelancet.com/journals/lancet/article/PIIS0140-6736(18)31928-7/fulltext.

Brackbill, Yvonne, June Rice, and Diony Young. 1984. *Birth Trap: The Legal Low-down on High-Tech Obstetrics.* St. Louis, MO: The C.V. Mosby Co.

Clarke, Adele E., Laura Mamo, Jennifer Fosket, Jennifer R. Fishman, and Janet K. Shim. 2010. *Biomedicalization: Technoscience, Health, and Illness in the U.S.* Durham and London: Duke University Press.

Conrad, Peter. 2005. "The Shifting Engines of Medicalization." *Journal of Health and Social Behavior* 46 (1): 3–14. DOI: 10.1177/002214650504600102

Corea, Gena. 1985. *The Hidden Malpractice : How American Medicine Mistreats Women.* New York: Harper & Row.

Dick-Read, Grantly. 1964. *Introduction to Motherhood.* London: William Heineman—Medical Books. Original edition, 1950. Reprint, 12.

Donnison, Jean. 1977. *Midwives and Medical Men.* London: Heinemann.

Ehrenreich, Barbara, and Deirdre English. 1989. *For Her own Good: 150 Years of the Experts' Advice to Women.* New York: Anchor Books and Doubleday.

Johnson, Candace. 2014. *Maternal Transition: A North-South Politics of Pregnancy and Childbirth.* New York and London: Routledge.

Katz Rothman, Barbara. 1982. *Giving Birth: Alternatives in Childbirth.* Harmondsworth and New York: Penguin Books.

Loudon, Irvine. 1997. "Midwives and the Quality of Maternal Care." In *Midwives, Society and Childbirth: Debates and Controversies in the Modern Period,* edited by Hilary Marland and Anne Marie Trefferty, 180–200. London and New York: Routledge.

Manderson, Lenore. 1992. "Women and the State: Maternal and Child Welfare in Colonial Malaya, 1900–1940." In *Women and Children First: International Maternal and Infant Welfare 1870–1945,* edited by Valerie Fildees, Lara Marks, and Hilary Marland, 154–177. London and New York: Routledge.

McCarthy, Niall. 2018. "Which countries conduct the most caesarian sections?" *Forbes,* June 23, 2021, October 15, 2018. https://www.forbes.com/sites/niallmccarthy/2018/10/15/which-countries-conduct-the-most-caesarean-sections-infographic/?sh=6c360fc218ea

Riska, Elianne. 2015. "Gendering the Medicalization Thesis." In *Gender Perspectives on Health and Medicine,* edited by Marcia Texler Segal, Vasilikie Demos, and Jennie J. Kronenfeld. Bradford, 59–87. Emerald Group Publishing Limited.

Tait Neufield, Hannah, and Jaime Cidro. 2017. *Indigenous Experiences of Pregnancy and Birth.* Bradford: Demeter Press.

3

THE SOCIAL CONTROL OF REPRODUCTION

Human reproduction is not determined by biological facts, as seen in theories of reproduction which are fluid and sometimes contradictory. Nor is how we reproduce determined by social facts, in other words that which is widely perceived as the normal social conditions for reproduction, today dominantly idealized as a family where the genetic contributors to the child, considered as mother and father, live together to raise the child. It is certainly the case that both biological aspects of reproduction and the social pressure as to how it should happen play very significant roles in how human reproduction is realized, but this is not the whole story. In sociology, social control is presented as a tiered process of informal expectations (family and immediate community expectations), norms, formal expectations (laws) and force that guide human behaviour. Contrary to popular belief, the overt threat of violence or legal sanction does not chiefly control social behaviour, but it is the internalized and intimately shared norms and the shame associated with their breach that most strongly impact how we act. The same can be said of the long history of social control of human reproduction where there are many evolving norms and tightly held beliefs that underlie and contradict formal controls of reproduction and parenting. The key debates within the social control of reproduction include who should be recognized as legitimate children and parents, and who has the right to control reproductivity, both at individual and population levels. Because of uterine pregnancy, and breastfeeding alongside the long-held association of women with child rearing, women are central to these debates. But not all women are equal socially speaking, and reproductive rights have never been the same for all women.

Increasingly, reproductive rights, which typically focus on the individual right to choose within formal structures of law, are being replaced by the more expansive concept of reproductive justice where intersecting social processes such as poverty and racialization come into play in understanding how reproduction

DOI: 10.4324/9780429467646-4

is enabled and constrained. For example, as chiefly white, middle-class women led reproductive rights movements during the 1960s seeking access to safe and effective contraceptives and abortion, Afro-American women in the US also sought access to social equity alongside men through the civil rights movement in part to provide the means and social stability to raise their families. These women's struggle was complicated by the intersection of race, class and gender. Although the pressure from the 1960s reproductive rights movement in most developed countries allowed women access to contraception and abortion, less was achieved in terms of reproductive justice for all. Women living in risky situations because of their race, their ethnic background, their class and their geographic location globally had to weigh their reproductive choices far differently than white women with access to economic resources in politically stable environments. And although today there is more attention given to reproductive justice, widespread and systemic injustices remain that restrict women's access to reproductive choice. Also, especially in the US, reproductive rights recognized in the 1960s and 1970s are now under attack, and those who suffer the most from claw back of legalized reproductive choice are women from marginalized groups.

Reproductive rights and social control – dominant historical trajectories

We have evidence at attempts to control human reproduction from as far back as 3000 BCE. In the ancient Egyptian text, the *Kahun Papyrus*, there are descriptions of how honey, leaves and lint could be combined and pressed into the vagina to block the passage of ejaculate into the womb. The *Book of Genesis* in the Bible speaks of the withdrawal method as a conscious act to avoid pregnancy in the story of Onan and Tamar. Other ancient contraceptive methods included crocodile dung and acacia gum pessaries (compressed matter placed in the vagina at the cervix that would block and repel sperm). A Roman bronze pessary dates to 200 BCE, and contraceptive sponges and condoms made from animal skins and intestines, fish bladders and linen sheaths were in use in ancient Egypt (about 2000 BCE); the contraceptive effect of breastfeeding was also known at this time. An early form of a gold IUD (intrauterine device) was used in the 1880s, and the Industrial Revolution introduced vulcanized rubber as a material for condoms. Many of these methods were effective and some continue to be used today: Acacia gum is a known anti-spermicidal and is used in modern preparations as such. Condoms continue to be used worldwide by 189 million men, making up 21% of contraceptive use as reported by the UN for 2019. IUDs, which still include metals such as copper for its anti-spermicidal qualities, were used by 159 million women (24% of all contraceptive use). The Pill makes up 16% of all methods used globally, but the largest type used is female sterilization at 26%. What this brief history of reproduction demonstrates is how long we have sought to control it and also the extent to which we do today: 854 million people in 2019.

Initially abortion was also considered a post-coital form of contraception. Herbal abortifacients date back to ancient Egypt and were used along with various instruments and massage to expel the early embryo from the uterus. Later, chemical means including caustics and other agents were directly applied to the uterus, and others were developed into pills and tinctures and sold to women to "regularize" or bring back their menstrual cycles. For many centuries, abortion did not carry the moral and political weight that it does today.

The Pill, a hormonal contraceptive, although not the most commonly used contraceptive today, has a significant social impact in European, North American and some Asian countries by making effective contraception widely available to women. The development of the Pill relied both on scientific developments in the understanding of human hormones and the persistence of especially two birth control activists, Margaret Sanger and Catherine McCormick, to create an effective oral contraceptive available for women to control their family size. Sanger, a long time US activist battling against the American Comstock Law (1873) that equated contraceptive information to pornography and outlawed its dissemination, encouraged Gregory Pinctus (a researcher in reproductive physiology), John Rock (a Harvard-trained infertility specialist and devout Catholic), and Min-Cheuh Chang, a Chinese-American reproductive biologist, to develop the Pill. Sanger engaged her friend McCormick (the second woman to graduate from MIT and who married into the wealthy family owning International Harvester) to fund the research into hormone-based contraception and its development into the first effective oral contraceptive. The US Planned Parenthood network grew out of these two women's collaboration and functions today to disseminate contraceptives and contraception information and to provide abortion. The Pill's effectiveness as a contraceptive – currently rated at 99.7% – and its relative ease of use (a daily oral pill), along with the timing of its release in the 1960s when strict religious and moral codes surrounding heterosexual activity were either relaxed or ignored on a large social scale, helped trigger the so-called sexual revolution.

Prior to the 1960s sexual revolution, reproduction was closely monitored and socially controlled by a range of norms and legal sanctions determined by a long history of Christian, Judaic and Muslim religious beliefs that placed the nuclear, heterosexual family as the proper and unique place for sexual activity and reproduction. Strict applications of Christian belief led to the outlawing of contraception around the turn of the 20th century in the US and Canada, and to powerful moral stances against contraception in many other industrialized countries. Yet at the same time, varied pressure from feminists, communists and socialists, as well as those interested in controlling the growth of designated populations for eugenic and economic reasons, helped develop effective and accessible contraception as "family planning."

Contraceptives, chiefly condoms, associated with prostitution (a long-standing vibrant business throughout Europe and North America), were referred to as the mechanical means of contraception and were carefully distinguished from family-planning contraceptives. So-called natural means of contraception, such as knowledge of women's fertile periods in their monthly cycle or the rhythm method, were part of early acceptable attempts at modern birth control. The Pill, chiefly because of its origin in science and its dissemination through medicine, was aligned with natural and acceptable modes of contraception. Even the Catholic Church briefly entertained accepting it alongside the rhythm method.

The pressure to develop acceptable, effective and available contraception and to provide access to safe abortion arose out of dire circumstances, especially for poor women. With industrialization came waves of immigration to cities starting in the early 1800s in western Europe and continuing well into the 20th century in North America and Australasia. The relatively sudden urban intensification alongside the sociopolitical effects of industrialization concentrated class difference in ghettoized areas of the city. The social control of reproduction followed. Working-class fathers in these ghettos were prone to underemployment and labour exploitation, leaving their families at great risk due to squalid living conditions, hunger, malnutrition and untreated illness and disease. Alongside these material conditions making "another mouth to feed" extremely challenging, were so-called moral activists, such as Anthony Comstock in the US, who managed to parlay strict religious beliefs of proper reproductive and sexual behaviour into social norms and law. In Great Britain, the same arose out of Victorian-era sensibilities surrounding sexual activity – male homosexuality and prostitution were outlawed – and social expectations tied women to religiously sanctioned and noble calls of marriage and motherhood – in that strict order. The medical historian Barbara Appleby finds that before the 1920s, many Christian churches (including both Catholic and protestant sects) relied on a theory of natural law dating back to the teachings of Thomas Aquinas to argue against contraception. Basically, the theory goes, the human body and its organs were designed by God for heterosexual reproduction; to interfere with this design was not only immoral but sacrilegious or going against the word of God. Sexual desire, with woman as the usual object of such, ran the grave risk of altering God's plan. In general, both Islam and Judaism traditionally held heterosexual marriage as the only divinely sanctioned place for reproduction, but their religious influence on secular society and its laws in most industrialized nations was limited by the marginalization of Muslims and Jews there. Ironically, these two large, organized religions did not adopt the Christian theory of natural law to argue contraception as sacrilegious and typically allowed it as long as it was used within marriage. Meanwhile the wedding of strict Christian belief with social control severely hampered the development and dissemination of safe and effective contraception making family planning near impossible, especially for women without the means to learn about and purchase effective contraceptives illegally. It also led to widespread exploitation of women who found themselves "in trouble" with a pregnancy outside of marriage.

A healthy industry in the form of homes for unwed women was established to deal with those women who strayed from the path of moral reproductive (in other words, sexual) decency. Many religious and other socially concerned groups ran such homes, especially in North America, Australia, New Zealand and Europe. Here women who had become pregnant (and clearly had unsanctioned heterosexual intercourse) were typically hidden from public view throughout their pregnancy, gave birth and, shortly afterwards, relinquished their newborns to adoption. The weight of shame and exploited labour involved was significant: many of these young women had to work hard at these houses to support the costs of their stay and as punishment for their moral slip. The Magdalene Laundries (asylums) in Ireland run by the Catholic Church since the 1700s until late in the 20th century provide an infamous example. The social historian Frances Finnegan reveals the abuse of women there, which led to a national enquiry and a formal state apology in 2013, with state compensation provided to the living survivors. Houses for "fallen women" and unwed mothers were common in newly expanding urban centres and were designed to maintain the appearance of reproduction as limited to properly married couples, firmly blaming illicit reproduction on women. The children born in these houses also secretly built proper families for infertile married couples (it is only relatively recently that adoption has been made a more open process). The stigma of pregnancy outside of marriage was great, and often young women went to such places with little resistance or right of reply. The surrender of their children to adoption was also inevitable, with little to no consent from the birth mother. The mass burials of tiny bodies often found at these homes raise questions of profound neglect and infanticide, including at some of the Magdalene asylums in Ireland, and at the Ideal Maternity Home in Nova Scotia, Canada, where butter boxes served as caskets. Today in the US, 49 states legally allow child marriage which has historically been used to "deal with" unwanted teen pregnancies, including having the girl marry her rapist. A study by the American organization devoted to ending forced and child marriage, Unchained at Last, estimates there were almost 250,000 child marriages in the US between 2000 and 2010.

Under such coercive and shame-bound conditions, women were quick to grasp that controlling their family size mattered a great deal to them and their families. There is evidence that throughout the 1800s and into the 20th century, women exchanged among themselves what information they could gather about effective contraception, at considerable risk to themselves. The historian Angus McLaren and the sociologist Arlene Tigar McLaren unearthed a 1930s letter from a Saskatchewan woman to her friend discussing home-made vaginal spermicides: "I don't believe she used it and I didn't either because it contains alum [a caustic agent] and I am scared to death of alum. It's as bad as caustic...." The use of condoms and diaphragms made from the newly manufactured vulcanized rubber during the 19th century throughout Europe and urban North America effected significant and, for many nationalists, disturbing drops in population growth – legal or not, obviously many were using contraception. The backlash to dropping birth rates included legal bans in Europe and North America on the distribution of contraception and contraceptive information rationalized by moral concerns that sexual desire was overtaking especially women's reproductive and domestic responsibilities, as well as by nationalist arguments that lowering birth rates would stunt economic growth. Doctors, increasingly more powerful as keepers of medical knowledge, tended not to share what they knew about conception and contraception, partly out of adherence to social mores (religious and nationalistic) and to laws against contraception, and partly to maintain their growing monopoly over medical information and practice.

Three distinct groups with differing reasons were interested in effective and large-scale contraceptive use. The first group including women led by the early 20th-century reproductive control activists Sanger in the US and Stopes in the UK saw the control of reproduction as essential to the complete liberation of women (alongside winning the right to vote). The second group focused on restricting certain populations, including the growing numbers of impoverished people in urban centres and the physically and mentally "unfit." Relying on terms such as "degeneracy," "mental sanitation" and "human damaged goods," some physicians around the 1900s concerned themselves with the protection of the future of the human race and national economies through sterilization. Paul Weindling describes how in 1895 the German physician and eugenicist Alfred Ploetz coined the term "racial hygiene" to address the declining German birth rate and the increasing number of mentally ill and disabled people in state institutions, all as economic concerns. At this time, things such as intelligence, crime, alcoholism and divorce were seen as genetically determined. In the 1930s, the Nazi party took "race" in Ploetz's theory of racial hygiene to represent the dominant Aryan race, and created genetic registries and blood banks to prove membership in the Aryan race and to justify elimination of anyone considered a pollutant: Jews, gypsies, homosexuals, people with disabilities, and mental "defectives." The Holocaust both relied on and helped develop reproductive and genetic theories of the time.

The sterilization of the so-called mentally unfit was also widespread in non-Nazi Europe and North America; in the same year that Nazi Germany passed its race laws (1928), the Canadian provinces of British Columbia and Alberta passed laws allowing the forced sterilization of mentally ill and "retarded" people. The Alberta Sexual Sterilization Act was repealed in 1972 after almost 5,000 people were sterilized under it. In 1906, the Eugenics Educational Society (now the Galton Institute) was formed in Britain to further "eugenic teaching and understanding in the home, in the school and elsewhere." It worked from the presumption that reproducing along so-called good and healthy gene lines would be to the benefit of society. It helped draft the 1913 Mental Deficiency Act, which rejected sterilization of the feeble minded but called for their social segregation. Between 1890 and 1920, the US states passed legislation to enforce sterilization in the feeble-minded, those with epilepsy, the intellectually disabled and the mentally ill. The laws were pitched as measures for social progress. As Angus McLaren and Anne Tigar McLaren state, "It was a cruel irony that many of the eugenically-minded doctors who opposed the family limitation of the 'fit' were clamoring for the forced sterilization of the 'unfit.'"

The third group interested in contraception were left-wing political groups and were studied by the social historians McLaren and Tigar McLaren in terms of reproductive politics. Although socialist parties in Europe and North America initially supported contraception at the turn of the century as a path to working-class emancipation through the elimination of poverty associated with large family size, the *Socialist Standard* in Canada published in 1930 an analysis of contraception as a tool of capitalism that could control labour supply and place the responsibility for eliminating poverty on the shoulders of the poor. Those making such arguments were aware of the forced sterilization laws of the day and saw such widespread and state-managed birth control as a menace. The Canadian Communist Party, also initially in favour of contraception as a form of protection for motherhood, changed its position in 1929 and criticized the birth control movement as a bourgeois enterprise that distracted attention from class struggle; both Stopes and Sanger were indeed upper-middle-class women working in poor communities. McLaren and Tigar McLaren conclude that the dominant masculine culture in the working class nursed romantic sentiments of heading traditional large working-class families and viewed new contraceptive methods as unnatural and not of their class. Meanwhile, many working-class women remained very interested and involved in controlling their family size.

A similar pattern is found with a fourth group interested in birth control: those racially inscribed as inferior. Afro-Americans also identified the public acceptance of contraception as a potential menace to their population. Although slavery had been outlawed since the Civil War, what followed can hardly be called emancipation. The contemporary American essayist Te Nahisi Coates explains how the US remains a deeply racially divided place, where the ability to own property, rates of incarceration and violence at the hands of the police, access to healthcare and employment equity remain racially determined. He tracks this divide from the time of the brutal plunder of African slaves' bodies, families and their labour, to the immediate clawback of Afro-American's right to vote following emancipation through poll taxes and lynching, through the systemic restrictions of their right to own property through real estate red lining, to today's mass incarceration rate which, according to the National Association for the Advancement of Colored People (NAACP), has African Americans imprisoned five times more than whites. As with the socialists and communists in the 1920s, those fighting for Black civil rights in the 1960s, especially male members of militant arms of the movement, came to see the largely white middle-class birth control movement as an attempt to reduce and control Black American populations.

Sanger and Stopes made the connection between family planning and poverty, reducing the matter to family size. Their reasoning ran that if women had the knowledge and ability to control their family size, they could lift their families out of poverty. The Black women's liberation movement made up of mostly working-class women and women on welfare sought protection for motherhood through welfare rights and access to decent housing and education. Unlike the white reproductive rights movement, the Black women's liberation movement focused not on the body but on the body politic. This tension in reproductive rights remains today, especially in the contradictory geopolitics of birth control where poor nations identified with large birth rates are targeted for mass birth control programmes by associations funded by industrialized nations responsible for the negative ecological effects of mass consumption. Both the African American women's liberation position in the 1960s regarding birth control and more recent critics of global population control programmes gave rise to the concept of reproductive justice.

In the meantime, contraception has become an acceptable practice around the world, with most industrialized nations lifting legal prohibitions around the late 1960s. The United Nation's Population Division reported in 2020 that of 1.1 billion women of reproductive age worldwide, 851 million are using some form of contraception. Significant variations occur: contraception use is 85% in China, the UK, the US and Canada but only about 15% of women in Angola, Benin, Mali and Somalia were using any form of contraception. The stigma associated with pregnancy outside of marriage has also relaxed considerably, especially in developed nations. According to the Organisation for Economic Co-operation and Development, in 2014 the rate of children born out of wedlock in Chile, Costa Rica, Iceland and Mexico was about 70%, while in Canada, the US and most European countries about 40% (in Greece, Israel, Turkey and Japan, it was less than 10%). The countries with high rates have seen the rates shoot up in the last 50 years (roughly coincident with when the Pill became available and the sexual revolution began).

With abortion, social control remains far tighter than for contraception. As stated earlier, abortion has not always carried the moral weight that it does today, especially in US politics and among certain Christian religious sects. Central to the contemporary debates surrounding abortion is the definition of human life and its moment of origin. We know that conception as understood today results from relatively recent developments in reproductive theory. This development involved the ability to see and to understand microscopic gametes (the egg, and sperm) and the early embryo, all of which are normally deeply hidden inside human bodies and are difficult to watch in action. Relying on animal models, we learned a lot about conception and early embryo development in mammals throughout the 19th and 20th centuries. In 1965, Lennart Nilsson's photograph of an 18-week-old human embryo blazoned the cover of the very popular photo magazine, *Life*, and sold 8 million copies in the four days following its publication. The image was used three years later in the major motion picture, *2001 – A Space Odyssey*, as an emblem of human potential. It was made using a very small lens on the end of a lit tube, an endoscope, a medical tool that had just started being used in medicine to visualize various body cavities and vessels requiring only small incisions. Nilsson took photos of a live four-month-old foetus inside the womb, exposing it to public view for the first time. Today, a variety of photographic techniques assisted with computer imaging can capture the moment the sperm are permitted entry through the egg's zona pellucida or egg covering, the first cell division of a fertilized egg, and the days-old cellular blastocyst attaching to the mother's womb lining. Commonplace in the medical management of pregnancy now are realistic computer assisted ultrasound images in the mother's uterus of the developing foetus, revealing details as small as eyelashes and tiny fingernails. Foetal pharmacology and fetal surgery are available in most developed countries. And genetically we now know more than ever before about how genes are exchanged during human reproduction and we have developed ways to engineer that process. All of these developments over the past 50 years have generated a tension between those who claim moral guardianship over the embryo and foetus as God-given people, those who wish to access and control embryonic and foetal development including reproductive physicians and geneticists and the woman growing the foetus and typically bearing the brunt of daily responsibility for the person born.

These multiple claims over the foetus colour the mechanisms of its social control. But this was not always the case. First-trimester (the first three months of pregnancy) abortions have long been sought and to varying degrees secured. Early abortifacients (materials that bring on the expulsion of the foetus from the uterus, usually at an early stage of pregnancy) included herbs, sharp instruments and massage or pressure applied to the uterus. In the *Ramayana*, an ancient Indian epic text (first appearing about 600 BCE), abortion is mentioned as practised by barbers to save the life of a pregnant woman. This position on abortion is often justified by an understanding of pregnancy in terms of "the quickening" or the time in the pregnancy when the pregnant women feels the foetus move inside of her, or what Sarah Knott describes as "the first certain sign of being pregnant." This concept developed long before hormone assays and computer-assisted ultrasound came into practice. For centuries, many, including Christians, considered this point in the pregnancy, normally occurring between the fourth and fifth month of pregnancy, as the moment of conception. Before this time, the prospects of the foetus were not certain, and indeed this is the time when spontaneous abortion or miscarriage typically occurs. Just as using various methods to prevent pregnancy were accepted early on, so was the discontinuation of pregnancy until the foetus was felt moving within the womb. And terminating a pregnancy to save the pregnant woman was also acceptable over two and half thousand years ago.

In the 19th century, as with contraception, social norms surrounding abortion shifted; it was rendered a significant threat to the natural order of reproduction and was considered immoral and made illegal. The UK first criminalized abortion in 1803, France in 1810, Australia in 1861, Canada in 1869, in Germany in 1871 (when it became a country this year) and in the US it was criminalized state by state around the turn of the 20th century. Initially the influential British law recognized the quickening principle, allowing for women to "regularize" their menstrual cycles in the first trimester. The quickening principle was dropped in 1837, and women aborting their own pregnancies were criminalized alongside abortionists in 1861. Despite these legal roadblocks, there continued a healthy commerce in the mail-order business of tablets and tinctures to "regulate" women's menstrual cycles, and hundreds of physicians were charged with the crime of committing an abortion. McLaren and Tigar McLaren refer to a complaint by Judge Winchester of Toronto in 1908 that hardly a week went by without a doctor being so named in the crime.

As the contraceptive pill was made commercially available in the 1960s, and legislation barring contraception was dropped in most developed countries, abortion was also decriminalized, but in fewer countries and with notable restrictions that reflected a bowing to religious, especially Christian, authorities. Typical laws from this period allowing abortion forced women to appear in front of hospital panels to make the case that their mental and/or physical health was in jeopardy if they continued with an unwanted pregnancy, or to go through mandatory state-approved counselling, which continues in Germany and the US today. In some places, the limitations remain extreme, allowing abortion only in cases of incest and rape. In Ireland (and ironically Northern Ireland which is politically a part of the UK) and parts of Latin America abortion remained strictly prohibited until the early 2020s, even if the life of the pregnant woman was at stake. It remains strictly prohibited in the Dominican Republic, El Salvador, Nicaragua and the Holy See.

With modernity, what were long considered private matters among women, including contraception, pregnancy, birth and the termination of pregnancy, were widely and decisively moved into the public realm where they were strictly regulated. Initially religious authorities assumed formal control over these reproductive moments; then, as medical science and practice gained moral authority over the mind and body, physicians became significant players and eventually functioned as the moral arbitrator over life. It is difficult to account for how many women have been maimed and killed in desperate attempts to control their troubling and shame-bound reproductivity. Home-based abortion techniques used by Canadian women at the turn of the 20th century ranged from placing the feet in hot water, to turpentine and carbide douches, to using lead pencils, knitting needles and crochet hooks to dislodge the well-embedded embryo in a blood-rich uterine lining. How many women died as a result of bungled, backstreet and self-induced abortions? It is very hard to tell. Such deaths were often reported by coroners as naturally occurring maternal mortality, sometimes to protect the woman's family, sometimes to protect a doctor involved. McLaren and Tigar McLaren make a careful estimation from reported maternal mortalities that between 1921 and 1946 in Canada, 4,000–6,000 women died from botched abortions despite there being a safe medical procedure available since the turn of the century.

But women did not take this lying down. As calls for civil rights and nuclear disarmament hit the streets throughout North America, Europe and beyond in the 1960s, so did women's right to reproductive control. The women's movements of the 1960s were largely focused on reproductivity partly because of its impact on women's ability to fully participate in a public sphere of work where pregnancy and children did not normally belong, but mostly to wrest back control over their bodies including reproduction and abortion. As explained above, not all women took part or were included in this movement. Afro-American women were forced to see the problem differently due to entrenched socio-economic racism. Also, abortion was lumped in with contraception by Black, male-dominant activist groups as white-orchestrated genocide of Black peoples. None of this deterred Afro-American women's interest in controlling their reproduction, including access to contraception and abortion, but racism made the matter more complicated.

"Our bodies, ourselves," "pro-choice," "keep your laws off of my body" and "if men could get pregnant, abortion would be a sacrament" are common slogans stemming from the 1960s reproductive rights movement. They emphasize two things: reproductive matters are both private and political, and control of reproductivity is primarily the control of women. This movement, which continues today due to constant pressures to reel back reproductive rights – chiefly abortion in the US – is characterized as a matter of choice by those in favour of a woman's right to choose her reproductive status versus a matter of morality by those who believe that no one should interfere with God-given reproductivity. In the US, arguably the world's most developed nation and one founded on principles of democracy and human rights, the right to abortion is described in terms of a war. Here all reproductive rights are ruled state by state, even though the precedent-setting Supreme Court case, Roe v Wade (1973), made access to abortion a constitutional matter of every American women's right to liberty of the person. In Alabama, abortion is almost completely banned under the 2019 Human Life Protection Act, which recognizes all unborn children as persons and allows for abortion only when the foetus is stillborn or when the pregnancy presents a serious risk to the life of the woman, which must be affirmed by a physician first. There are no exceptions made for cases of rape or incest. Other states, including Georgia, Mississippi, Louisiana, Missouri, Kentucky and Ohio, have recently replaced the quickening principle (when a pregnant woman feels the foetus move) with "heartbeat" provisions (externally detecting the heartbeat with instruments) to limit abortion. In 2019 in Georgia, a month after Governor Brian Kemp signed a heartbeat abortion ban, lawyers for the American Civil Liberties Union, Planned Parenthood and the Centre for Reproductive Rights, and lawyers for the state filed a suit challenging the law. These heartbeat abortion laws limit abortion up to six weeks (when an electric muscle pulse can be detected in the tissue that will become the heart) even though many women do not know they are pregnant at this stage. In June 2021 Texas passed its heartbeat abortion law, which was upheld by the Supreme Court the following September. Some American states have also adopted "management" measures in abortion clinics, effectively chipping away at Roe v Wade, forcing patients through days' long waiting periods and required "counselling" sessions, some of which attempt to mislead women into associating abortion with cancer, serious mental health outcomes and infertility. Many abortion clinics operating in these states do so under duress, with no local doctors willing to suffer the consequences of being known as an abortion provider, by constant picketing by anti-abortion protestors who harass patients and health providers, and with violence. In 2015, *The New York Times* reported that at least 11 people had been killed in attacks on abortion clinics in the US. Meanwhile, criminal cases of foeticide brought against pregnant women are on the rise in the US, where women suffering from miscarriage and stillbirth have been charged with murder.

This war, argues the sociologist Carol Joffe, is also between "the two Americas of reproductive health." There is one population that is typically urban, educated and with the means of securing access to effective contraception on a regular basis, and to safe abortion without question. And there is the other America populated by those living in rural areas, in poverty and with less chances for higher education, who do not have the means to pay for, or to access, contraception and abortion services. These two Americas also fracture along racialized lines. And the final irony: when asked in a 2017 survey, most women in the US seeking to terminate a pregnancy said they do so for financial reasons – they cannot afford to raise a child or another child –leaving those the most in need of family planning as the least likely to get it.

Globally, access to legal abortion varies, but there are trends in some South American countries similar to the situation in the US to strictly limit abortion access. The Professor of Law Michelle Oberman describes that unlike the earlier history of botched abortions that relied on home-made instruments (the infamous coat hanger, for example), self-administered dangerous chemicals and back-alley practitioners with little medical training and no regard to sterile technique and follow-up, abortion access has recently been transformed by the abortion pill: RU 486 or mifepristone. Administered properly, this normally prescribed medication is 98% effective, and the rare cases of excessive bleeding or incomplete abortion that may result can easily be treated by a doctor without evidence of an abortion attempt. In El Salvador where in 1998 abortion was completely banned, the abortion rate did not drop as women accessed mifepristone through the Internet. What Oberman also discovered was that doctors under the 1998 legislation were recruited to police women's reproductivity, including cases of suspected self-induced miscarriage/abortion despite being unable to prove if vaginal bleeding or miscarriage was a result of using mifepristone or not. Poor women and girls were criminalized as a result. In a country where both public and private healthcare are available, Oberman discovered that out of 129 prosecutions of women and girls for illegally attempting to abort between 2001 and 2011, the majority of which were triggered by doctors' reports, not a single one came out of the private healthcare sector. Some of these cases involved women who had spontaneously miscarried and sought medical attention and were wrongly imprisoned for having attempted an abortion. When evidence of an early abortion attempt is difficult, if not impossible, to distinguish from a naturally occurring miscarriage, doctors effectively become judges as well as a form of reproductive police. Some publicly funded doctors were found not to report cases when they believed a woman or girl had made an abortion attempt, instead upholding their Hippocratic Oath to do no harm to their patient and to treat them medically to the best of their ability. However, patients who could afford private healthcare did not run the risk of policing and judgement by their physicians at all. An almost identical class-based discrimination occurs even in places where abortion is not criminalized, and in the US, it is complicated by race.

Today, women suffering spontaneous miscarriage in the US are also being caught up in the justice system in states where there are fetal infanticide laws combined with new legal provisions strictly limiting (just short of outlawing) abortion. And here too money matters. Money can buy you travel to a state with less stringent abortion provisions. It can allow you access to mifepristone over the Internet, and money usually furnishes women with the knowledge and confidence to self-administer the drug. This has for long been the case. Historically throughout North America, Europe and Australasia some doctors and coroners did not report botched abortions as such, either out of concern for the women or to profit from keeping quiet. Women with enough money could buy access to safe abortions either locally or abroad; doctors have known how to perform abortions safely since the turn of the 20th century. Women of means with access to paths of privilege could pay for confidentiality and freedom from persecution for illegal abortion. Up until the 1960s and 1970s and the legalization of abortion in most developed countries, a dilation and curettage (D&C) was a minor gynaecological surgery used to control excessive uterine bleeding following a miscarriage or from fibroids, which also served as a safe and masked form of abortion.

With the advent of re-restrictions on abortion and the recent move to criminalize alleged abortion attempts based on shaky evidence and effectively outside of court, Oberman's argument – what is happening in El Salvador will likely happen in northern and western countries as well – does not seem at all far-fetched. In places where national and state politics are heavily influenced by religious organizations focused on banning abortion, the procedure will continue to be practised, but secretly or out of state or country; it will be limited to those who can afford and access not only the drugs and safe procedures but also the cost of keeping the matter confidential. Medical practitioners will determine who will be reported for violations, and snitching on a woman's reproductivity could be opened to all around her. As big data are increasingly involved in managing medical information, especially for insurance purposes in the US private model of healthcare delivery, women's reproductive status could also be tracked and shared. This helps explain why recently there have been demonstrations, especially in the US, for women's reproductive rights featuring women dressed as the reproductive handmaids from Margaret Atwood's dystopian fictionalization in *The Handmaid's Tale* of a divided US in the not too distant future. In Atwood's telling, a part of the US has evolved into a fascist fundamentalist religious regime preoccupied with declining birth rates, and as a result, the regime strictly monitors and controls women's lives by class, caste and fertility. On May 4, 2019, two American anti-abortion organizations projected live ultrasound images of a third-trimester foetus in a womb on large screens in Times Square. Then in a full-page ad in the Sunday *New York Times* they advertised the event with people getting a chance to see the images on their cell phones. In the same year, California passed a bill requiring all state-funded universities to provide medical abortion (mifepristone pills) on campuses. There are a variety of fertility apps available where women can track when they ovulate, including Clue, Flo, Eve, Glow, Ovia and Sprout. Although these seem innocuous and even cute, the apps are prone to the same surveillance (sanctioned or not) and algorithmic treatment of personal data as any other.

The Center for Reproductive Rights, an international organization devoted to advancing reproductive rights worldwide, divides abortion law throughout the world into five categories: on request, on broad social or economic grounds, to preserve health, to save a woman's life and total prohibition. What is interesting is to compare these categories to how many women worldwide they affect: total prohibition = 90 million (5%) women; to save a woman's life = 359 million (22%) women; to preserve health = 237 million (14%) women; on broad social or economic grounds = 386 million (23%) women; and on request = 590 million (36%) women. Although the last category contains the largest group of women, the first three categories where abortion is totally banned or severely restricted affect 686 million women, that is, 41% of all women in the world. It is also important to note that gestational limits for abortion vary widely, from six weeks (Texas, Ohio, Georgia and Missouri, USA) to 24 weeks (the UK). The circumstances allowing for abortion also vary; for example, in the UK, there has to be medically determined risk to the life, or mental or physical injury to the woman or substantial physical or mental health risk to the child if born. The UK does allow for socio-economic harm to the family as an indication for abortion. What the numbers above reveal is that almost a third of fertile women worldwide cannot legally access abortion or can only do so if their life is determined to be at risk. And where this is the case is where access to contraception access also tends to be compromised.

And what about those who want to reproduce and are not allowed? Michael Warner in 1991 coined the term "heteronormativity" or the common and taken-for-granted social norms of heterosexuality including that children are properly born to married, heterosexual couples. Laura Mamo provides a reckoning of how lesbians in particular have managed to reproduce despite this social control of who should be pregnant and give birth but increasingly cannot without special assistance. Those who are married and heterosexual but cannot reproduce draw public sympathy and attention, and secret adoptions quietly normalized such families with others' children who were born out of wedlock. However, adoption in most countries where legislation for such exists was long denied to anyone not fitting the heterosexual, married norm, including single women, lesbians and gay men. It still is the case in many places such as all African countries except for South Africa, much of Asia including China and India, many Eastern European countries and Russia. Gay men were and continue to be impeded or banned from parenting due to widespread social smear tactics that equate a male homosexual orientation with pedophilia. This discrimination sometimes spills into legislation that prohibits openly gay men from teaching and otherwise being involved with children. Lesbians are not immune from similar treatment: their children have been removed from their care when their sexuality was exposed and treated as deviant. Today trans people are fighting for reproductive rights and proper medical support.

Becoming a parent and parenting is easier for homosexual women than for gay men, both socially and biologically. Initially both homosexual men and women hid their sexual preference behind heterosexual marriages of convenience and also became parents this way. As moral prohibitions against parenting out of wedlock dropped after the 1960s sexual revolution and women's rights movements, lesbians and single women in the UK, for example, began self-insemination groups. In San Francisco, the lesbian group, Daughters of Bilitis, held discussion groups on lesbian motherhood as early as 1956. The self-insemination process did not require medical assistance; it required only a willing sperm donor, tracking the ovulation period and a turkey baster. Women could also intentionally expose themselves to becoming pregnant without letting their male sexual partners know. The Sperm Bank of California opened in 1982 and was the first in the US to offer services to lesbian and single women; proper semen screening became crucial following the identification of HIV and its transportation in bodily fluids in the mid-1980s. For gay men, becoming a parent is more complicated as it not only requires a woman to agree to bear and give birth to a child she may not raise, but also requires legal manoeuvring to have a male sexual partner recognized as a legal parent and to perhaps remove the birth mother's parental rights. Many of these barriers, in addition to widespread discrimination and stigmatization, apply to trans people seeking to create families. Despite all of these barriers, there are places that support queer family formation: San Francisco, long a centre for promoting homosexual and now bisexual, transsexual and nongender-binary rights, has a well-established system of services, legal and medical, to help create families outside of the heterosexual norm.

Reproductive justice – the social determinants of reproductive health

The shift from a rights to a justice perspective in the social control of reproduction is a move away from formal measures of control of individual bodies, typically laws, to broader concerns of social justice including the right to sustainable living – including food and safe shelter, public safety, education, employment – and the right to cultural or community expression or belief. Family planning and control over one's reproductivity and sexual practices are understood within the context of these things. In her history of the US reproductive rights movement from the point of view of women of colour, Jennifer Nelson demonstrates how Black women transformed the movement from one of reproductive rights to reproductive freedoms. The term reproductive freedom was used in a 1979 statement of the Committee for Abortion Rights AND Against Sterilization Abuse or CARASA (*author's emphasis*) and refers to an array of freedoms far more expansive than individuals' access to contraception and abortion. This array includes the freedom from social discrimination and the policies that arise from such that can simultaneously prohibit "undesirable" people from reproducing through forced sterilization and an effective control of welfare-dependent Black and Hispanic populations. Nelson argues that contemporary efforts to secure reproductive freedom must come from the bottom-up and move away from the limitations of "choice" as individual women deciding whether or not to be pregnant and bear children. Women marginalized by their race and ethnicity combined with systemic poverty often find themselves trapped within policies that target their reproductivity as a cause of their problems and do little to address the broader issues of systemic discrimination and structured economic inequalities. This holds true not only in the US, but among racialized and indigenous populations in most other developed countries, as well as in populations throughout the so-called developing world.

Global population programmes started in earnest following the Second World War and are premised on two basic concepts. The first is neo-Malthusianism, which states that the world's limited carrying capacity is threatened by quickly expanding populations, especially in developing countries where birth rates are typically among the highest worldwide. The second concept is that development – understood as economic and social stability – requires controlled population growth. In the early 1800s, the world's population reached 1 billion; in the 1930s it reached 2 billion, in the 1960s 3 billion and in 2020 it almost reached 8 billion. It is this demographic trajectory that inspired global population planning by groups such as the US-based Population Crisis Committee (PCC), which was created in 1965 and which continues today under the less threatening name, Population Action International. The PCC was instrumental in creating the Office of Population within the US Agency for International Development (USAID), the United Nations Fund for Population Activities (now the UN Population Fund or UNFPA) and the PCC assisted in fundraising for International Planned Parenthood. All of these groups share a perception that population growth is a significant threat to the future of humanity, and that the problem lies chiefly in underdeveloped countries.

The first national population control programme started in India in 1951 following US President Lyndon B. Johnson's refusal of food aid to the country when famine threatened, due to a perception that the country would do nothing to address their growing birth rate. To answer initial suspicion among the so-called Third World countries about First World control of their populations, the message was changed to "a call in the name of humanity for the sake of the entire planet." Distancing population control programmes from any single government by running them through the UN helped to sell the idea, and family planning became a powerful sign of progressive societies. By the 1970s, other countries joined in with instituting national family planning policies, including developed countries such as Japan, Norway, Sweden and the Netherlands.

The challenge in many developing countries, was, and continues to be, the lack of infrastructure for delivering safe and effective methods for family planning. Initially this was seen chiefly as a problem of getting the right means of fertility control to large populations. Vertical systems of delivery were typical where government officials passed birth rate targets and budgets down to regional authorities who distributed contraceptives and providers to local centres, often through medical clinics. These vertical delivery systems tended to engage in misleading and coercive measures at the local level to meet regional and national targets. In Bangladesh for example, the non-governmental organization (NGO), UBINIG, discovered that women were being sterilized in exchange for bags of rice and saris when food and clothing were scarce. Although population control programs did help some in establishing healthcare networks and in distributing western-style medical care in economically dependent countries, these healthcare delivery systems and the people using them were also exposed to unethical drug testing, a practice that according to the NGO investigating the activities of multi-national corporations, SOMO, continued into the 21st century. Population control programs have also been criticized as misguided and self-serving in the targeting of impoverished populations by wealthy populations which lead to the 1994 official end to population programs at a UN sponsored Cairo conference. Population targets, and the incentives and disincentives used to meet them were banned, and in their place arose an expanded definition of health and wellbeing, especially for women and girls, that included education on fertility and contraception. Many development strategies in underdeveloped countries engage with this education-based model alongside programs designed to make effective contraceptives (including long-lasting ones) more readily available. This despite the fact that the annual growth rate of the globe's population has halved from 2% to 1.08% since the late 1960s. Although the actual number of people still grows each year, it does so at a slowing rate: the UN predicts that it will take until 2057 for the global population to reach the 10 billion mark.

Do underdeveloped countries deserve the continued attention they get in terms of population control programs? Since the inception of these programs in the mid-20th century, concern for the environment and consumption have entered the equation. Initially, underdeveloped nations were also blamed for environmental degradation: coal use, deforestation for fuel, poor sewage management, pollution of water ways, and so on. In the 1970s Paul Ehrlich, the population scientist famous for publishing *The Population Bomb*, and John Holdren, a scientist concerned with environmental change and energy who later served as President Obama's senior advisor on science and technology, argued that deteriorating environmental conditions (typically understood as pollution in the 1960s and 1970s) were caused by three factors: affluence (A), population (P), and technology (T). This generated the formula to measure rates of environmental impact

(I) as I = P + A + T, commonly referred to as IPAT. Ehrlich and Holdren gave the greatest weight to population. The left-leaning and feminist environmental policy scholar, H. Patricia Hynes, pointed out in 1993 how developing countries are chiefly associated with the population variable, while developed nations are responsible for most of the affluence and technology figures. She saw the need to distinguish within the affluence variable between those who consumed luxury goods versus those who consumed to survive. She also argued to include military technology (MAT) and its significant polluting effect. This rendered a different formula: I = (PAT)survival + (PAT)luxury + MAT. Then she called to recognize the effect of environmental support and conservation (which then typically came from small and local groups) as C: I = C − (PAT)s + (PAT)l + MAT. She concluded that to indicate the lack of women's agency in virtually every variable, P should stand for patriarchy. Her main point, compatible with the reproductive justice approach, is not to lay blame for degradation of the planet due to exploding populations at the feet of women, especially poor women.

In various explorations of maternities and modernity in Asia and the Pacific, Kalpana Ram and Margaret Jolly argue how dominant ideals of maternity within a Eurocentric view of linear development are attempts to re colonize or neo-colonization. For example, in post-independent Malay, mothering becomes an individualized activity among an array of state-sponsored programs by promoting maternal health according to a western medicalized model and a newly focussed attention by the state on the child and her welfare. These moves to modernize (westernize) and develop nations relies on the construction of a split between old (traditional, rural, extended family mothering, home health) and the new (modern, western, nuclear family mothering, medicalized maternity and infant care). Newly self-governing, formerly colonized countries adopt the split and work to bring their populations up to a level of development like those in the West. The formal social control of reproduction, from conception to raising a child to adulthood, is a key part of the process, and follows dominant notions of development. Whereas what especially women experience in the processes of maternity and modernization is more complex and based on shifting meanings as both traditions and the medicalization of birth are questioned and adapted. The ideology of reproductive care and child wellbeing as social progress is also active in marginalized populations within so-called developed, western countries.

In 2015 the Canadian government accepted the federally sponsored Truth and Reconciliation Commission's Report as a way of addressing the country's treatment of Indigenous people through enforced residential schooling that was designed to wipe out their cultures and language and exposed over 150,000 children to horrific treatment, including forced separations from family, community and homeland, intentional starvation, and sexual abuse. The last federally run residential school was closed in the late 1990s. Another, and often hidden aspect of Canada's treatment of Indigenous people, is the forced sterilization of Indigenous women especially those from remote and northern parts of the country, which led to a Saskatchewan-based class-action lawsuit in 2019. Based on research by Karen Stote, the suit alleges sterilizations without women's consent occurred as late 2018 throughout Indigenous populations in Canada. Stote describes the widespread practice as an act of genocide as well as colonization. Up until 1969 in Australia, Aboriginal people especially mix-raced children, were removed from their families under the White Australia Policy (1901–1966) in the hopes that their Indigenous bloodlines would be "washed" out as their genetics were absorbed into a white genetic pool. Referred to as the "stolen generations" these children are often compared with the Indigenous children forcibly placed in Canadian residential schools. Aboriginal girls in Australia were encouraged to marry white men in order to physically "whiten" the population and eventually eradicate the Indigenous population. As late as 2018 the UN also called on Australia to abolish forced sterilization of women and girls with disabilities, as well as intersex people. These are all aspects of contemporary colonization through the lens of reproduction.

How we socially control reproduction also extends to pro natalist policies, or policies to encourage certain people to reproduce. Since the rise of the modern nation and nation-based global economics, low population rates have been a concern to the developed state. Western European birth rates dropped significantly following the First World War due to the war itself, as well as to rising interest in and the availability of the means to control family size. According to the World Bank, although the global birth rate rose after the Second World War to an all-time high of just over five children per woman in 1965, it has been dropping steadily ever since. By 2017 it dropped to under 2.5; North America, countries of the European Union, China, Australia and New Zealand, South Korea and Russia all have rates of 1.8 or lower. A rate of 2.1 is considered necessary for a stable, replacement population. Despite important variables to consider in measuring the impact of birth rates, including geo global location, impact of consumption on the environment, rising life expectancy, lower infant and maternal mortality rates, some countries have adopted pro natalist policies or strategies. They do so to stabilize or strengthen national economies, to address the imbalance between increasing aging populations and diminishing younger working populations, and to protect language, ethnicity, religion and national identity. In 1966 Romania prohibited abortion and created incentives for women to have children, including improvements to working conditions and maternity leave. Because France experienced a falling birth rate earlier than most other European countries with the advent of industrialization in the 1800s, it was among the first to create a pronatalist policy. Between 1920 and 1940 it rolled out a national education program directed at children and young adults about falling birth rates and their national impact under the direction of the National Alliance for the Growth of the French Population, and passed the pronatalist law, Code de la famille in 1939. In 1988 the Canadian province of Quebec put a pronatalist policy into effect to protect its unique French culture and language within the dominant English North American context. The policy included escalating, at-birth payments, a family allowance for all children under 18 years, and an additional allowance for children under six. The first of Singapore's pro natal policies to address one of the lowest birth rates globally (1.2) was in 1987, and were followed by revisions and enhancements in 2004, 2008, and 2013. In 2019 The Hungarian government announced pro natal incentives, including removing taxes, reducing credit payments, and increasing access to credit for mothers with more than three children. The Russian political leader, Valdimir Putin put a pronatalist policy in place in 2007 including an escalating cash incentive on the birth of each child, increased parental leave, and compensation for daycare costs. Increases to this policy were enacted in each of the following six years.

And in between population control and pro natalism lies a more complex management, chiefly by women, of the pressures social control brings to reproduction. In Canada the care of pregnant and birthing Indigenous women has finally started to come under criticism, for example by the Indigenous scholar and midwife, Karen Lawford for separating women from their families, communities and way of life as women are routinely evacuated thousands of kilometres to urban centres for medicalized birth and neo natal care. Now some modern medical contexts are welcoming Indigenous family and community members and their rituals into birthing rooms. While reproductive justice, including decent housing, clean water, Indigenous-controlled child welfare, and access to modern reproductive healthcare and education under Indigenous peoples' terms, form part of continued demands by many Indigenous communities across Canada within a heightened awareness of abuses and neglect of Indigenous people through welfare and medical systems as well as by Residential Schools. Tamil women on the coast of southern India struggle with both the impact of a longstanding caste system and criticism from modernized westernized medical practitioners for the backward ways of their midwives. As the Tamil scholar who works among these people, Kalpana Ram states, "the project of reform... is not only an emanation of colonization but also bears certain important continuities with much older precolonial forms...". And yet, these women work to evade the negative impacts of both pre and post colonialism by shifting their religious practice to Christianity to escape the negative effects of the caste system, and by sustaining their communities through traditional activities including fishing, trading and local midwifery despite and sometimes in conjunction with westernized medical care and standards of childrearing.

The social management of identity also plays a role in the control of reproduction, especially in terms of social justice. We have seen how many countries interested and engaged with eugenic ideals adopted policies to improve national populations since the turn of the 20th century, culminating in the widespread horrors of the Shoah. The Nazi program in the 1920s and 1930s to ethnically cleanse the German population of Jews also included people with disabilities, homosexuals and those without a permanent claim on the land (gypsies). A considerable portion of western developed nations adopted eugenic policies to inhibit birth rates among the disabled (those considered mentally and physically unfit) allowing forced sterilization. In the UK male homosexuality has long been outlawed, one way or another, from 1533 to 1967 (lesbianism was outlawed in 1921) and initially punished by death and "cured" in the 20th century by chemical castration. Gay, lesbian, bisexual, trans sexual and nongender binary people continue to be formally and informally persecuted in places throughout the World: In Russia, the motivation for increasing its population rate arises out of the typical concerns for a stable internal economy, as well as out of Putin's conservative, homophobic nationalism. This has led to the Russian Orthodox Church joining forces with the state in promoting "family values" and in restricting reproduction to heterosexual and married couples, and outlawing homosexuality. The battle for reproductive rights for LGBTQ2+ people has only emerged recently and typically in places where their sexual identity is legitimized and protected. Finally, migrants, especially undesired immigrants, continue to be read as problematic in terms of their numbers ("wave" is a common description of them as a group). Many developed nations are formally and actively reducing or refusing their entry into local populations as a perceived threat to the reproduction of the ideal state.

Paternity claims and paternity rights, or the rights of fathers, have long formed a significant part of the social control of reproduction by identity, as they intersect with patriarchy and the powerful norm of heterosexuality. The historian, Nara Milanich has produced a comprehensive history of the continual hunt for certain paternity from Ancient Roman law to Internet-available DNA paternity kits. According to Roman law, *Pater semper incertus est* (the father is always uncertain), *mater certissima est* (the mother is always certain), and therefore, *pater est quem nuptiae demonstrant*, or the father is whom the marriage identifies. And so, as Milanich states, paternity is always embedded more in socializing fictions than biological fact, and that "the quest for the father [is] deeply politicized, culturally fetishized, and now thoroughly commercialized." Despite the surety that today's DNA testing promises, paternity remains more than a biological link, and even genetic markers are not always certain. The political philosopher, Mary O'Brien, bent the Marxist theory of historical materialism – or how we make sense of ourselves socio-politically in the material world – to feminist analysis. As maternity is usually certain (although with the advent of new reproductive technologies, this is less the case), and paternity has long been uncertain, O'Brien describes paternity as a social fiction generated to protect male interests and to inject some paternal certainty into the picture. All children born of a heterosexual, sanctioned union were of the husband as indicated by the globally common paternal surnaming of children and in the determination of inheritance rights and privileges. This is how men leave their mark historically, whereas women mark their time through the birth of their children, which forms an intimate and certain relationship with regeneration and with history.

Milanich demonstrates that even when obvious signs of racial difference are used to challenge paternal claims, other considerations carry more weight, as in Italy when inter racial children were born of white Italian mothers and the Black American soldiers liberating Italy in the Second World War. Despite strong public opinion that such "mulattini" or mixed children were obvious signs of women's infidelity and Black men's sexual predation and aggression, Italy's need to centre the family in re-righting the nation after the war (a position shared by both the socialist government and the Catholic Church) turned away from obvious fact. In the famous case of the "little Moor of Pisa," Antonio Cipolli, despite being born with what many around him, most notably the husband of his mother, considered Black features (dark skin and curly hair) and proof of his mother's infidelity with one of the Black soldiers from the nearby American base, the courts eventually appointed the husband, Remo Cipolli, as the legal father, and so named the child out of protection of the nation's interest in preserving the family as a pillar of social stability, no matter what the biological paternity.

Another side of hidden paternity is the exploitation of it by those who control artificial insemination or AI. AI has been part of medical practice since the turn of the 20th century and involves inseminating women, thus bypassing hetero-sexual coitus as a way of becoming pregnant. The process allows for any sperm to be used, and in cases where in a married heterosexual couple the male was in-fertile, donor sperm was used. Elizabeth Yuko explores the ethical ramifications of the first reported case of successful AI with donor sperm, which was in 1884 by an American doctor who used the sperm from a medical student considered the best looking of the class. The woman inseminated was unconscious for the procedure and was unaware that she gave birth nine months later to a child bi-ologically unrelated to her husband. The husband was informed by the doctor, William Pancoast. And later, the 25-year-old son was informed of his biological parentage by one of the former medical students present at the insemination just before he published his account of the insemination in 1909. Sperm donation has since become an international, multimillion-dollar business typically controlled by legal protection of donors from paternal responsibility for custody and inher-itance to any biological offspring. It is also now a typically open medical practice in that inseminated women, their partners and often the offspring are aware that the social father (he who the marriage indicates) is not the biological father. But hidden paternity also persists. It can be the intentional choice of women seeking to become mothers without the biological father involved in the rearing of the child. It can be the result of shame associated with a pregnancy that results from rape and sexual assault, including incest. And it can be a result of contemporary malpractice by doctors.

Sarah Zhang and Jacqueline Mroz independently report on how regularly cases arise where doctors who practice AID (artificial insemination by donor) do not rely on the careful management of donor sperm through registered sperm banks, but supply the donated sperm themselves, giving rise to public moral outrage, to uncertain genetic lineage with potential health implications, and to interbreeding minefields especially when the communities are small. In 2019 the Ontario fertility doctor, Norman Barwin, had his license revoked for insemi-nating 11 women with his own sperm, while a court case in the Netherlands involving the fertility specialist, Jan Karbaat, finally released evidence following his death in 2017 that he was the biological father of 49 children. In the 1980s, the American reproductive specialist, Cecil Jacobson, was found to be genetically related to 15 of the children of his patients seeking fertility treatment, while the Indiana-based doctor, Donald Cline, was found to have fathered at least 48 children through his fertility clinic between 1979 and 1986. Notably in this last case, the court found no criminal wrongdoing nor any human rights breech in the practice; only professional misconduct for deceiving his patients. In 2019 the state made such malpractice illegal, while in Texas, Eve Wiley, the biological daughter of her mother's fertility doctor there, is advocating that such practice be considered criminal sexual assault. During the atrocities of the Bosnian War between 1992 and 1995 up to 12,000 Muslim women were raped, chiefly by Serbian fighters. Not only was this considered torture of the women by the International Criminal Tribunal for the former Yugoslavia, it was also identified as a Serbian-sanctioned attempt at ethnic cleansing through forced insemination, which was used intentionally by the Serbs to disrupt Muslim communities as a Muslim woman pregnant with the child of a Serb risked rejection from her community along with her child.

Today, Milanich points out, paternity testing is more accurate and commercially available than ever before. A van containing a mobile DNA testing unit with the loud proclamation on the side, "who's your daddy?" has been trolling New York City's neighbourhoods since 2012. DNA fingerprinting, central to forensic identification in both real and the many fictionalized accounts of criminal investigation, was originally developed in the 1980s for paternity testing, and is now offered online for about $80 USD, as well as by New York's ice cream truck-like DNA testing van. Interest in DNA fingerprinting for paternity has spread worldwide from the US: the company EasyDNA offers Internet kits with mail-in testing in 39 countries, while the UK-based website Nimble Diagnostics explains paternity testing today in 36 languages. The service is also available from Chinese and Indian companies. And what is this information serving? DNA fingerprinting is used by governments and courts to help decide in custody and child support cases, as well as to determine immigration and citizenship claims, including the recently state-sanctioned denaturalization of citizens. There is not much public interest in fictionalized investigation series exploring these applications of paternity (and now maternity) testing. Paternity and its tricky status have long been wrapped up in the social control of reproduction of the family, from individual cases of alleged infidelity to the reproduction of the state and the geopolitics of migration.

Conclusions

The social control of reproduction is complex. It pulses constantly from the intimacy of individual families through medicalized reproductivity to state and global imperatives and protections. It reinforces existing inequities between peoples distinguished by race, sexuality, income, religious belief and so on. It is simultaneously the restriction of undesirable populations – usually characterized as unproductive economically, a threat to the environment and global safety, and often brown or black – and the promotion of others –normally characterized by economic wealth, high consumption and education rates, and whiteness. And in between, people manage to assert their reproductivity despite impediments: women create self-help insemination groups, gay men and lesbian women swap reproductive capacities to help each other form families outside heteronormativity, women in former colonized contexts step carefully between tradition and modern medicalization to get what serves them and their children best, and some doctors aid women in controlling their reproductivity despite legal sanctions. Reproduction is not always controlled through the passage of laws, and not all laws protect all people's reproductive rights. Reproductive justice does not look the same everywhere, and it is not the same for everyone.

Further reading

Appleby, Brenda Margaret. 1999. *Responsible Parenthood: Decriminalizing Contraception in Canada*. Toronto: University of Toronto Press.

Atwood, Margaret. 1985. *The Handmaid's Tale*. Toronto: McClelland and Stewart.

Balcom, Karen. 2002. "Scandal and Social Policy: The Ideal Maternity Home and the Evolution of Social Policy in Nova Scotia, 1940–51." *Acadiensis* 31 (2): 3–37. ISSN:0044–5851.

Bashford, Alison, and Philippa Levine. 2010. *The Oxford Handbook of the History of Eugenics*. Oxford: Oxford University Press.

Bongaarts, John. 2020. "United Nations Department of Economic and Social Affairs, Population Division World Planning 2020: Highlights." *Population and Development Review* 46 (4): 857–858. DOI: 10.1111/padr.12377

CBC News. 2019. "Fertility doctor's licence revoked after he used own sperm to inseminate patients." Accessed 19 November 2019. https://www.cbc.ca/news/canada/toronto/fertility-norman-barwin-disciplinary-hearing-1.5183711.

Center for Reproductive Rights. 2021. "The World's Abortion Laws." Accessed 26 June. https://maps.reproductiverights.org/worldabortionlaws.

"Child Marriage – Shocking Statistics." Accessed 6 July 2018. http://www.unchainedatlast.org/child-marriage-shocking-statistics/.

Coates, Ta-Nehisi. 2018. *We Were Eight Years in Power: An American Tragedy*. New York: One World Publishing.

Ehrlich, Paul. 1968. *The Population Bomb*. San Francisco, CA: Sierra Club and Ballentine Books.

Finnegan, Frances. 2004. *Do Penance or Perish: Magdalen Asylums in Ireland*. Oxford: Oxford University Press.

Foster, Diana G., M. Antonia Biggs, Lauren Ralph, Caitlin Gerdts, Sarah Roberts, and Maria Glymour. 2018. "Socioeconomic Outcomes of Women Who Receive and Women Who Are Denied Wanted Abortions in the United States." *American Journal of Public Health* 108 (3): 407–413. DOI: 10.2105/AJPH.2017.304247.

Hynes, H. Patricia. 1993. *Taking Population Out of the Equation: Reformulating I=PAT*. Amherst, MA: Institute on Women and Technology.

Joffe, Carole. 2009. *Dispatches from the Abortion Wars: The Costs of Fanaticism to Doctors, Patients, and the Rest of Us*. Boston, MA: Beacon Press.

Karen, Stote. 2015. *An Act of Genocide: Colonialism and the Sterilization of Aboriginal Women*. Halifax: Fernwood Publishing.

Knott, Sarah. 2014. "Early Modern Birth and the Story of Gender Relations." *History Workshop Journal* 78: 287–294. DOI: 10.1093/hwj/.

Lawford, Karen, and Audrey R. Giles. 2012. "An Analysis of the Evacuation Policy for Pregnant First Nations Women in Canada." *AlterNative: An International Journal of Indigenous Peoples* 8 (3): 329–342.

Mamo, Laura. 2007. *Queering Reproduction*. Durham: Duke University Press.

Mclaren, Angus, and Arlene T. McLaren. 1986. *The Bedroom and the State: The Changing Practices and Politics of Contraception and Abortion in Canada, 1880–1980*. Toronto: McClelland and Stewart.

Milanich, Nara. 2019. *Paternity: The Elusive Quest for the Father*. Cambridge, MA and London: Harvard University Press.

Mroz, Jacqueline. 2019. "Their mothers chose donor sperm. The doctors used their own." *The New York Times*, August 21, 2019. Accessed 20 November 2010. https://www.nytimes.com/2019/08/21/health/sperm-donors-fraud-doctors.html.

Nelson, Jennifer. 2003. *Women of Color and the Reproductive Rights Movement*. New York and London: New York University Press.

Nilsson, Lennart, Linda Forsell, Lars Hamberger, and Gudrun Abascal. 2020. *A Child Is Born*. 5th ed. New York: Random House.

O'Brien, Mary. 1981. *The Politics of Reproduction*. Boston, MA: Routledge & Kegan Paul.

Oberman, Michelle. 2018. *Her Body; Our Laws: On the Front Lines of the Abortion War. From El Salvador to Oklahoma*. Boston, MA: Beacon Press.

Ram, Kalpana, and Margaret Jolly. 1998. *Maternities and Modernities: Colonial and Postcolonial Experiences in Asia and the Pacific*. Cambridge: Cambridge University Press.

"See for yourself." (Advertisement). 2019. *The New York Times*, May 5, 11.

Smietana, Marcin, Charis Thompson, and France Winddance Twince. 2018. "Making and breaking families—reading queer reproductions, stratified reproduction and reproductive justice together." *Reproductive Biomedicine & Society Online*, June 26, 2021. https://www.ncbi.nlm.nih.gov/pmc/articles/PMC6491795/#bb0285. DOI: 10.1016/j.rbms.2018.11.001.

The World Bank. "Fertility rate, total (births per woman)." Accessed 2020. https://data.worldbank.org/indicator/SP.DYN.TFRT.IN.

United Nations Department of Economic and Social Affair. 2020. Contraceptive use by method 2019-data booklet. Accessed 25 June 2021. https://www.un.org/development/desa/pd/sites/www.un.org.development.desa.pd/files/files/documents/2020/Jan/un_2019_contraceptiveusebymethod_databooklet.pdf.

Warner, Michael. 1991. "Introduction: Fear of a Queer Planet." *Social Text* 9 (4 [29]): 3–17.

Weindling, Paul. 1993. *Health, Race and German Politics Between National Unification and Nazism, 1870–1945*. Cambridge: University of Cambridge Press.

Yuko, Elizabeth. 2016. "The first artificial insemination was an ethical nightmare." *The Atlantic*.

Zhang, Sarah. 2019. "The fertility doctor's secret." *The Atlantic*. Accessed 26 June 2021. https://www.theatlantic.com/magazine/archive/2019/04/fertility-doctor-donald-cline-secret-children/583249/.

4

REPRODUCTION AND SEXUALITY

The relationship between human reproduction and sexual desire has long been socially mediated. Undoubtedly the introduction of morally acceptable, legal, effective and widely available contraception starting in the mid-20th century followed soon after by lifting of restrictions on abortion in many developed countries had wide-reaching social impacts on human reproduction. For the first time since prehistoric cultures worshipped a feminine divine as fertility, reproduction was split from heterosexual intercourse: this type of sexual activity did not have to result in pregnancy. Heterosexuality began to be publicly challenged as a powerful social norm that had long confined sexuality to only married men and women and that assumed women were natural at child-rearing and confined them to the home. Allowing for the planning of parenthood in the second half of the 20th century helped women to work outside the home in record numbers. Young people around the world joyfully formed the 1960s' sexual revolution liberating heterosexual desire from shame and the binds of matrimonial-sanctioned sex. Then, gradually, gay rights advanced, eventually including the call for reproductive rights for non-heterosexuals as deeply rooted definitions and practices of kinship continued to be challenged. And throughout this period, money is to be made: hormone-based contraception has been a big pharmaceutical-based business that seeks new markets with the possible suspension of monthly menstruation and the medicalization of male sexuality.

Unhinging reproduction from heterosexuality

Family planning pioneers Marie Stopes (UK) and Margaret Sanger (US) helped start a worldwide movement at the start of the 20th century that allowed women to decide if, when and how often they would be pregnant by calling for widespread distribution of contraception and contraceptive information that until this

DOI: 10.4324/9780429467646-5

point was widely illegal and often considered amoral. This was no small feat and is clearly laid out in the social historian Elaine Tyler May's history of the Pill. Not only did this movement have to address the medical monopolization of knowledge at the turn of the 20th century which extended to understanding the particulars of human reproduction including knowing when women were fertile in the monthly cycle and what could prevent sperm from meeting and combining with the egg. Laws prevented this information from being distributed out of moral concerns: the US Comstock Laws prevented the distribution of contraceptive information as pornographic, a legacy from the historical association of contraception with prostitution that was widely shared throughout western Europe, North America and Australia. Stopes and Sanger shifted the moral debate to poverty and socio-economic well-being. They argued that planned family sizes would allow those living in poverty to move up economically. Their strategy was to place clinics in poor neighbourhoods where they initially dispensed contraceptive information and built up women's confidence to assert their reproductive choice at home, ostensibly only those married to men.

Decades later came the development of an effective contraception without the historical contamination of prostitution practices: the Pill. Due to the fundraising and organizing efforts of Sanger, the hormonal contraceptive was developed and made available to women as patients (not impoverished citizens) by the early 1960s. Sanger succeeded in securing the funds required and brought together willing scientists and a physician to make it happen. In May 1960 the US approved the Pill for medical release; in 1961, 400,000 women were taking it, four years later the number jumped to over 3 million and in 2019, the UN estimated that 151 million women worldwide used the Pill as contraception. Although not the cause of the sexual revolution, the Pill certainly played a key part as the risk of unwanted pregnancy was significantly reduced by the effectiveness of the drug, and as a physician-controlled medication, it was distanced from the legacy linking contraception with prostitution. The widespread uptake of contraception in the 1960s not only required the technical means for safe and effective control of pregnancy, it required a relaxing of moral and legal restrictions on individual, especially women's, reproductive control. The reproductive rights movement that arose in most industrialized nations – democratic, socialist and communist – reflected a turn towards the rights of women away from the sanctions of chiefly large, organized religions who had long held positions of authority over human reproduction. But increased medicalization of women's reproduction, including contraception, left women contending with medical authorities over their reproductive choices.

The sexual revolution was more than the means to control reproduction; it was also a move to liberate sex from shame under the main slogan of the movement: "free love." Premarital sex throughout much of the 20th century and in most developed countries carried significant shame. So-called "unwanted pregnancies" and the centuries-old cottage industry in homes for unwed mothers are testament to the power of that shame. The ability to enjoy heterosexual sex

without the threat of pregnancy was a great release and was felt widely throughout a politically active and resistant middle class, chiefly in white college culture
in North America, western Europe and Australasia, while women in socialist and
communist states including the USSR and China were not only granted access to
contraception but also to safe and widely available abortion.

Foundational to this newly won heterosexual freedom are two significant
social movements and growing unrest internationally. The first is the US-based
civil rights movement starting in the mid-1950s and lasting well into the 1960s
which was led by Afro-Americans demanding the realization of the freedom and
rights promised to them by the Emancipation Proclamation of 1862, but which
instead was followed by a brutal and persistent racialized regime. The second was
the women's liberation movement during the 1960s and 1970s which focused on
securing reproductive rights (to contraception and abortion), sexual liberation,
equal access to work and fair pay and gaining political influence generally. Both
movements occurred during heightened criticism of especially American influence in geopolitical conflicts and the growth and dissemination of capitalism
globally. Notable protests included the Kent State University protest against US
involvement in the Vietnam War where American troops fired on and killed
their own citizens, and the May 1968 uprising of university students alongside
labourers in Paris. The world was changing, and government authorities were
being challenged by their own, relatively young populations of reproductive age.

Notably absent from these demonstrations, protests and civic actions were
those seeking an end to the stigma and abuse associated with homosexuality.
Although gay men and lesbians (the chief components of non-heterosexual identity at this time) were certainly present and to some extent were forming their
own social groups, they remained largely hidden from public view, including in
protest, until the Stonewall Riots of 1969 in New York City. Stonewall is the
name of the Greenwich Village club where gay men, lesbians and drag queens
met to socialize, usually with protection from police interference by the mafia
who owned and profited from the bar (unlicensed), which featured extremely
watered-down drinks and virtually no attention to hygiene provisions including clean washroom and running water behind the bar to wash glasses. Gayle
Pittman provides an artefact-based history of gay life in New York City, leading up to and including the riot that became a watershed for gay rights in the
US and beyond. On June 28th the bar was not warned of an impending police
raid and 13 patrons and employees were roughly rounded up and arrested while
cross-dressing patrons' sex was checked by police in the bathrooms. Patrons and
others living nearby reacted violently and forced the police, a few prisoners and a
local journalist to take refuge in the club as rioters outside tried to burn it down.
The riot was quelled with no one seriously hurt, but it has since become known
as a galvanizing force that led to the US-based gay rights movement: the days of
being holed up in substandard closets and always vulnerable to police brutality
were coming to an end for those who defied the heterosexual norm. In 2016,
President Barack Obama designated the area surrounding the Stonewall Inn as

a national monument to gay rights. Although this movement did not initially address reproduction, it would have been very difficult without it to assert reproductive and parenting rights for members of the LGBTQ2+ communities, especially gay men and transgender people.

Donald West and Richard Green bring together a significant collection of international comparisons of sociolegal developments in homosexuality. Lesbians' struggle for sexual-based identity rights was typically not the same as that of gay men. This had to partly do with patriarchal assumptions of what constituted sexual acts. For example, in a long history of addressing non-heterosexual activity from the Roman conquest of Britain to Victorian England, only male-to-male sexuality is addressed: King Henry VIII passed the Buggery Act in 1533 making homosexuality between men punishable by death. The Act was repealed in 1861, and replaced in 1885 by the Criminal Law Amendment Act banning sexual acts of "gross indecency" between males, which expanded the definition of criminal sexual behaviour among men beyond buggery. Only in 1921 did the British Parliament extend sexual gross indecency to females, and in 1956 recognized sexual assault between women as a crime. Cross-dressing and passing as the opposite sex have long been practised in the UK and elsewhere, sometimes with deadly consequences – the cross-dressing Englishman, Kenneth Crowe, while wearing his wife's wig and dress, was beaten and strangled to death in 1950 by a boxer John Cooney when he found out Crowe was not male. Sexual confirmation surgery in Britain started in the 1930s, but transgender people remained deeply closeted throughout most of the world until the 2010s. A similar trajectory of severe legal prohibitions against especially male homosexuality is found throughout the world and persists in places such as Russia and some African countries. Also, violence, harassment and discrimination against non-heterosexuals continue despite some legal recognition of LGBTQ2+ rights, most notably the right to marriage.

Not only was non-heterosexual desire criminalized for a long period and remains so in various places worldwide, establishing legally recognized non-heterosexual kinship has virtually been impossible. As with the UK, throughout the 19th and 20th centuries many developed countries established laws defining and protecting marriage as a heterosexual union and the proper place for reproduction and the raising of children: the creation of kin. It was not until the late 20th century that the gay rights movement, combined with lesbian, bisexual and trans groups and then later with queer and two-spirited associations, formed what is commonly referred to as the LGBTQ2 community. Today those refusing or questioning a dualistic approach to gender, those who are androgynous along with a growing number of forms of gender expression are indicated as LGBTQ2+. Although hardly a single community, the collaboration between non-heterosexual interest groups in many developed democracies globally has helped secure sexual and reproductive rights beyond the dominant male–female dyad. Between 2001 and 2020, same-sex marriage was legally recognized in 27 countries, including in the UK in January 2020. Earlier, legal recognition of same-sex couples, parenting and reproductive rights were only possible through a heterosexual masquerade: gay men and lesbians would marry and have children legally recognized through the marriage. Even if they eventually divorced their opposite-sexed partners, gay people's sexual orientation had to remain hidden in order to maintain their parental rights; so-called sexual deviance and obscenity are powerful legal tools used to remove parental rights. Prior to the 1970s, adoption was also limited to married, heterosexual couples. Today, same-sex couple joint adoption is allowed in 27 countries. However, the legal recognition of same-sex marriage and all the rights and privileges that come with marriage such as inheritance, insurance as well as parenting continue to be a struggle in many parts of the world.

Kinship unhinged

The public recognition of the Stonewall Inn as a national monument to gay rights marks a significant progression from the 1885 UK criminalization of male homosexuality as buggery and other legislative bans on sexual practices. But there is continued persecution of LGBTQ2+ people such as the US Orlando gay night club shooting in 2016 that left 49 people dead and 53 seriously hurt. Today, in many African countries and in Russia where homosexuality is criminalized, the punishments for violating heterosexual norms are harsh and violence against LGBTQ2+ people is on the rise even in places where it is legally protected. On the other hand, significant LGBTQ2+ rights have increased in places including in the US, Canada, the UK and most of western Europe. Notable among these are the right to reproduce. As contraception marks the major shift in the relationship between sexuality and reproduction for modern heterosexuals, conception and the making of queer families marks what sexuality and reproduction mean for homosexuals and trans people. The American queer studies scholar Elizabeth Freeman takes this a step further and argues that the origin of the so-called modern family is at the intersection of *kinship* (how relatedness is recognized and practised) and sexuality, which allows us to tie together sex and reproduction in radical new forms.

Freeman asks whether non-conforming sexually identifying people actually change the rules of kinship when they seek the same structures as those in place for heterosexuals: naming and rearing children in dyads of parents who are legally responsible for the child, limiting state and financial support to legally recognized couples and so on. Is the answer to restricted access to kinship to expand membership to include gay and lesbian fathers and mothers or to get rid of the clubs based on the kinship model of heterosexual, nuclear families? Or is it more complicated? Freeman traces queer theory to the French philosopher Michel Foucault's characterization of the history of sexuality as a "regime of sexuality" that emerged in the 19th century and managed in many ways (legally, morally, medically) the meaning of sexual desire and experience: the criminalization of buggery, the casting of especially gay men as perverse and ungodly and categorizing homosexuality as a mental illness. Freeman argues that this regime, however, sits apart from a regime of "alliance" or kinship, which controls matrimony and legally sanctioned reproduction.

What, asks Freeman, would a regime of queer affinities or kinship look like? Queering or radically twisting the structure of kinship is not limited to the LGBTQ2+ community, although the feminist philosopher of sexuality Judith Butler does ask if "kinship is always already heterosexual?" With both questions, Freeman and Butler are acknowledging the powerful social effect of assumed kinship norms: the heterosexual dyad of parents raising children expected to be genetically related to the parents and to each other. In Canada the power of this norm was tragically expressed in the so-called 1960s "scoop" of tens of thousands of Indigenous children from families deemed unfit to raise them. Reasons for removal of these children from their families, their communities, their language and their culture included perceived infractions of the kinship code: children sharing beds with siblings and adults other than biological parents such as aunts, cousins and older children taking responsibility for raising the children. The scoop relates to what Freeman calls affinities over space: we can recognize others, including LGBTQ2+ people, in normal kinship roles such as mother, father, parent and partner, but not beyond to menages a trois, quatre, or cinq, friends as parents, or raising children in cliques, communities and tribes. Normal affinities or kinship also span time in prescribed ways. We can recognize children of gay or lesbian parents when they are adopted from the generation below, but what if that rule of descent is not obeyed and contradicts "normative generationality?" Why do we have difficulty grasping the concept of adults adopting each other in parenting and child roles?

The radical reformation of kinship or the social recognition of who relates to whom also relies on socio-technical developments in reproductive and sex-trait hormones, called the "pharmaco-pornographic regime" by the philosopher of the science of sexuality, Beatriz (now Paul) Preciado. Preciado paints a picture of a "post-industrial, global and mediatic regime" emerging after the Second World War that includes the medical coining of the term gender and the discovery that any child's sex can be changed up to 18 months (1947), and the first demographic study of "sexual deviation" (1941). In 1953, Hugh Hefner begins publication of the first North American pornographic magazine, *Playboy*, to be distributed alongside daily newspapers; Marilyn Monroe is featured nude on the front cover. The 1972 pornographic film *Deep Throat* becomes the most watched film of all time and helps launch a multibillion dollar industry in porn. In 1941, natural molecules of progesterone and oestrogen are distilled from the urine of pregnant horses, and soon after are synthesized and mass produced for the contraceptive pill, and for "treating" transsexualism during the 1950s and 1960s. Following several failed attempts at physically managing penile erectile dysfunction, the vasodilator drug Sildenafil (commercially known as Viagra) was approved for treatment in 1988. As Preciado states, "the political management of body technologies that produce sex and sexuality can be seen to progressively become *the* business of the new millennium." And this sexual regime is assumed as heterosexual.

When the North American psychiatrist John Money coined the term gender and differentiated it from biological sex in the late 1940s, it was part of the wider regime of normalizing, celebrating and profiting from the sex industry described by Preciado. But first feminists in the 1970s and then early queer theorists seized on the plastic term to challenge sexism ("the exaltation of masculine labour and domestic maternity)," heterosexism and the persecution of homosexuality. With increasing pressure from homosexual rights groups and a progressive psychiatric subgroup, homosexuality was declassified as a mental illness in 1973 (although a decade later "gender identity disorder" or transsexuality was added in as a disorder). Between the 1970s and 1980s, lesbians formed self-insemination groups in San Francisco and London, UK, while other women continued to fight for control over their reproductivity (on-demand abortion, for example) and for equitable, paid employment and childcare to allow them to work in the public domain. The relative stability of biologically based sex difference (now differentiated form the social construction of gender) is then challenged in the early 1990s with attempts to find the genetic determinants of sex. The sociologist of science and technology Joan Fujimura examines these studies and finds that they are based on and reproduce social assumptions of sexual difference: "Sex, even at the genetic level, is a sociomaterial process and product." Socially the challenge to sex and gender dichotomy occurs with the coming out of transsexuals and their calls for access to the pharmaceutical and surgical means to sex affirmation. Meanwhile, LGBTQ2+ people hijack new reproductive technologies designed to reinforce heteronormativity to generate different families. The following question remains: Do these discoveries and reformation of sex affinities represent a new and progressive kinship? Or as Mamo and Alston-Stepnitz ask, does this represent a repopulation of the same kinship structures with different actors that also perpetuates the commercialization of reproduction with new markets, as well as the exploitation of others through contractual surrogacy?

Capitalizing on reproduction and sexuality

In the early 2000s, contraception moved beyond the realm of family planning to the medicalization of lifestyle management. In December 2005, the Canadian national magazine, *Macleans*, featured a cover with the provocative statement: "The End of the Period – Menstruation Will Soon Be Optional." It was referring to the oral hormone-based contraceptive pill used as a way of reducing the number of times women menstruate during the year. Typically, women shed the lining of their uterus about once a month. When taking the oral contraceptive, the female reproductive system is effectively tricked into thinking the body is pregnant and therefore the necessary preparation of the uterine lining to accept a fertilized egg does not take place. Since its inception, the monthly pack of the Pill has contained seven placebo pills (differently coloured) and women are instructed to take these following three weeks of the contraceptive pills. By ceasing the pill with the active hormonal ingredients, a minor irritation in the uterus occurs and there is some bleeding as a result called a withdrawal bleed. This is not an actual period or shedding of the uterine lining when no implantation of a fertilized egg occurs. But it looks like one and is kept there to maintain the fiction of menstruation. The possibility of not bleeding at all has always been present with the Pill; many people who menstruate but would rather not typically because of work responsibilities, such as pilots, astronauts and surgeons, do not take the placebo pills but continue on with the contraceptive ones and never bleed.

Manufacturers of the Pill marketed this option to a much broader market than busy and heavily responsible professionals who may have found managing vaginal bleeding a significant hindrance to performing their duties. Seasonale is one such product released in 2003, and one of its ads features a young woman twirling carefree in her purple-dotted white dress, the dots falling to the ground around her. The ad explains that, "unlike other daily birth control pills, SEA-SONALE lets you have four periods a year." This leaves the woman free to enjoy: "disco.tango.hip-hop.nonstop." And presumably leaves men to enjoy sex with a rarely menstruating woman. In 2004, the pharmaceutical company Barr made $87 million selling Seasonale. The 2005 article in *Maclean's Magazine* raises the medical advantages of "menstrual suppression" and refers to the Brazilian gynaecologist Elsimar Coutinho, who in 1999 published the book: *Is Menstruation Obsolete? How Suppressing Menstruation Can Help Women Who Suffer from Anemia, Endometriosis, or PMS.* Here, it is pointed out how the modern woman, due to delay and limitation of childbirth, earlier onset of menstruation and a far lower maternal death rate than her 19th-century counterpart, experiences far more menstrual cycles: 400 for the modern woman compared to 50 for the 19th-century woman. And menstruation is blamed for making worse anaemia, migraine headaches, endometriosis and polycystic cysts. The conclusion: menstruation is a risk to modern women's health. The solution: suspend it through the constant medication of menstruating women.

The sociologist of medicine Jennifer Fishman tracks Viagra as the biomedicalization of impotence as medical attention in general shifted from life-threatening illness and disease to focus on life-limiting conditions, such as the medicalization of menstruation. Traditionally, impotence was accepted within the 19th-century medicine as an inevitable part of male ageing, a sort of biological winding down. We have seen how during the early part of the 20th century, the discovery of sex hormones and their relationship to sex traits, including penile erections, led to crude methods of distilling sex hormones (from slaughtered animals initially) to be used by physicians and others to reverse the effects of ageing, including sexual performance in men. Since then, the increased reliance on pharmacy in medical practice, the "molecular turn" in medical sciences, along with a struggle between psychologists and physicians to define and control the condition, transformed male impotence as an expected part of ageing into erectile dysfunction. This became a concern to men of all ages, and so medicalized male sexuality.

As pregnancy and birth were increasingly medicalized especially after the Second World War, Fishman tracks how sexuality became a significant part of medical and psychological research. Studies by the biologist and sexologist Alfred Kinsey (1953) and the gynaecologist William Masters and sexologist Virginia Johnson (1960s and 1970s) were landmarks in normalizing and bringing sexuality to the practice of medicine, providing typologies and pathologies and laying the ground for medical treatment. As we saw in the history of contraception, sexual activity, even in morally condoned arrangements such as heterosexual marriage, has long been hidden from public view and prone to slipping from its proper place with serious social consequences. Information about how to engage in heterosexual sex without the risk of pregnancy was illegal in the US when Kinsey released his report on the naturalness of human sexuality. In the 1950s, abortion was a deadly back-street activity, and children born outside of marriage were usually put up for adoption amidst the shaming and social ostracization of unwed mothers. To bring sexuality into medicine was a step away from the long moralist hold over sexual activity by dominant organized religions. As sexuality was recognized as a part of human health, notes Fishman, both mental and physical wellness and illness were attributed to sexual practices. And sexual discrimination received the stamp of medical authority: a year before Kinsey released his report, homosexuality was included in the first edition of the Diagnostic and Statistical Manual of Mental Disorders (DSM) as "paraphillia" (sexual perversion and deviation). Women's sexual desire hardly figured there. This left heterosexual male desire indicated by erectile function as the main cause of medical concern.

That (male) sexual performance is not only a physiological matter but a psychological one as well, gave rise to a territorial struggle over its medical management. Once sexology was on the table, sexual performance understood as male impotence (women's sexuality remained out of the picture until the 1980s) was treated in the 1970s and 1980s through talk therapy by sexologists, psychiatrists and psychologists. In the 1980s, urologists, physicians specializing in the urinary tract and the male reproductive system, became interested in the physiology of erections and the possibility of controlling them pharmaceutically. Fishman recounts the legendary moment when the urologist Giles Brindley injected his penis with phenoxybenzamine and allowed those attending his session at the 1983 meeting of the American Urological Association to inspect and examine his drug-induced erection. This opened the gateway to a host of injections, pumps and implants to address an unwanted flaccid penis. It also spurred criticism, such as that by the sex psychologist Leonore Tiefer, who in the 1990s described this medicalization of male sexuality as a way of normalizing phallocentrism, or the reduction of sexual pleasure to penis-based male desire. Ironically Tiefer is also credited with changing the term from "impotence" to "erectile dysfunction" in an attempt to destigmatize the condition.

Despite feminist criticism, urologists continued to explore methods to cure this emerging sexual dysfunction and were looking for something more natural than pumps, injections and implants. The oral contraceptive pill was lauded as a hidden method of contraception that would not interfere with the mood during sex, and was sold by one of its developers, John Rock, to the Catholic Church as a natural method of avoiding conception (contrasted to mechanical methods such as condoms). The same occurred with erectile dysfunction: It was presented as a medical way to extend erection-based sexuality into older age in a non-invasive manner. As with many pharmaceuticals, the drug that was to become Viagra was first developed by Pfizer for another purpose: treating heart angina (which also requires management of smooth muscle tissue and blood flow). Fishman outlines how Jacob Raifer, a urologist, and Louis Ignarro, a pharmacologist, who worked on nitric oxide in cardiology, also published in 1992 an article on how it managed the smooth muscle function of the penis, enabling erections. In 1998, Ignarro, along with several others, received the Nobel Prize for his work that identified the role of nitric oxide in the cardiovascular system. Pfizer capitalized on their development of sildenafil and released it as the erectile dysfunction drug Viagra the same year. By 2003, five years later, Viagra had earned Pfizer $7.4 billion. Typically, each pill costs $30 and $60, although some lower-priced, low-potency variations are now emerging (the US patent expired in 2020). Now the treatment of this relatively newly described dysfunction of male sexuality will be more accessible financially. Not only does erectile dysfunction reduce male sexuality to a single function of the penis while continuing to feed a phallocentric view of sex, it medicalizes male sexuality for men, young and old. And beyond medicine, it has become a significant component in maintaining a particular masculine lifestyle in the face of ageing, drug and alcohol abuse and social expectations of what constitutes male sexual desire.

Conclusions

Sex, sexuality and reproduction have long comingled in our societies over the millennium. For at least 2,000 years we have understood that there is a causal connection between heterosexual copulation, pregnancy and birth. What we have made of that connection has varied, and what we have done to manage that connection, especially in the last 50 years, is significant with important impacts on the socialization of sexuality and reproduction, especially in developed nations. First, we managed to prevent reproduction technologically with the advent of effective and widely available contraceptives, especially the Pill. Socially, there was a release of requirements to limit heterosexual sex to marriage, followed by a decriminalization of homosexuality and moves towards de-stigmatization of and anti-discrimination against non-heterosexuality. By the new millennium the release of sexual desire from bounds, heterosexual, homosexual and beyond, led to considerations of new reproductive contexts or kinship. The same pharmaceutical regime that grew since the Second World War to manage conception and sex trait expression for the heterosexual norm was hijacked to serve queer people in their gender affirmation and to help non-heterosexual families with having children. This regime also developed new norms of pharmaceutically managed femininity (suspended fertility and reduced menstruation) and masculinity (penile erection-focused sexuality available from youth to old age). And whatever the social norm, there were markets to be capitalized. The so-called new reproductive technologies entered the scene in the middle of all of this. Assisted conception medicine (as it came to be called as conception was next medicalized) quickly took up its place in the regime and grew into its own successful enterprise. It too was exploited not only economically, but by those seeking access to kinship outside of the heterosexual norm. It was also exploited for genetic research and application, leading to the establishment of a new regime: replication.

Further reading

Butler, Judith. 2004. *Undoing Gender.* New York: Routledge.

Fishman, Jennifer R. 2010. "The Making of Viagra: The Biomedicalization of Sexual Dysfunction." In *Biomedicalization: Technoscience, Health, and Illness in the U.S.*, edited by Adele E. Clarke, Janet K. Shim, Laura Mamo, Jennifer Ruth Fosket, and Jennifer R. Fishman, 289–306. Durham and London: Duke University Press

Freeman, Elizabeth. 2007. "Queer Belongings: Kinship Theory and Queer Theory." In *A Companion to Lesbian, Gay, Bisexual, Transgender and Queer Studies*, edited by George Haggerty and Molly McGarry, 295–314. Malden, MA and Oxford: Blackwell Publishing Ltd.

Fujimura, Joan H. 2006. "Sex Genes: A Critical Sociomaterial Approach to the Politics and Molecular Genetics of Sex Determination." *Signs: Journal of Women in Culture and Society* 32 (1): 49–82. DOI: 10.1086/505612.

Lee, Erica Vilet, and Tasha Spillett. 2017. "Indigenous women on the Prairie reproductive freedom." *CBC News.* Accessed 25 November. https://www.cbc.ca/news/indigenous/opinion-indigenous-women-reproductive-freedom-1.4418787.

Lianne, George. 2005. "The end of menstruation." *McLean's*, December 12, 2005, 40–46.

Mamo, Laura, and Eli Alston-Stepnitz. 2015. "Queer Intimacies and Structural Inequalities: New Directions in Stratified Reproduction." *Journal of Family Issues* 36 (4): 519–540. DOI: 10.1177/0192513X14563796.

May, Elaine Tyler. 2010. *America and the Pill: A History of Promise, Peril, and Liberation.* New York: Basic Books.

Pitman, Gayle. 2019. *The Stonewall Riots: Coming Out in the Streets.* New York: Abrams.

Preciado, Beatriz [Paul]. 2008. "Pharmaco-Pornographic Politics: Towards a New Gender Ecology." *Parallax* 14 (1): 105–117. DOI: 10.1080/13534640701782139.

Tiefer, Leonore. 2016. "The Viagra Phenomenon. Sexualities." *Sexualities* 9 (3): 273–294.

West, Donald, and Richard Green. 1997. *Sociolega Control of Homosexuality: A Multi-Nation Comparison.* New York: Kluwer Academic Publishers.

5

IN VITRO FERTILIZATION AND GENETIC ENGINEERING

In 1978, Louise May Brown, the world's first "test-tube" baby born using *in vitro* fertilization (IVF), came into the world. At the same time, most women in developed countries had become accustomed to giving birth in hospital with specialized doctors in attendance. Caesarian rates were on the rise and radical hysterectomies were common treatment of uterine fibroids in women. Effective contraception was legal and widespread in these same places, with abortion often legally available but typically in hospitals requiring approval by physicians. Gay men and lesbians were less closeted but still highly socially marginalized with no legal rights to form families; although some groups of lesbians organized self-insemination groups in London, UK, and San Francisco. The human genome had been identified for over two decades and geneticists had started exploring how to identify genetic-based disease. Reproductive hormones were used by gynaecologists and obstetricians on women in heterosexual couples who were unable to get pregnant; there was very little research in the area of male factor infertility. The average wage gap between Black and white American males was almost 30%. Caps limiting welfare according to restricted family size were in place in the US, and global aid was tied to reducing birth rates in the developing countries where rates were high. There was talk of creating a male hormone-based contraceptive to match the Pill, but nothing came of it. In 1964, four years after the Pill was approved by the FDA, the drug company Searle netted $24 million. By 1980, the pharmaceutical giant Pfizer indicated sales worth $2 billion primarily for the sale of antibiotics, but less than two decades later it made over $1 billion in a single year for the sale of Viagra alone. Genentech, the first firm to use human genes, was created in 1976, and by 1982 marketed the first recombinant DNA drug: human insulin. Obstetrics and gynaecology, like pediatrics, was low on the list of medical specialties compared to cardiology and neurology. But all of this was

DOI: 10.4324/9780429467646-6

going to change with the advent of a technology that brought human conception outside of the human body. IVF allows for human gametes (eggs and sperm) and very early conceptuses with complete and unique genetic codes to be transferred, examined and engineered.

But what seems drastically new in reproductive medicine and human genetic engineering is not so in reality. In order to understand the significance of IVF in humans as a threshold to so-called new reproductive technologies, we need to link it to previous applications in animal husbandry, to the development of reproductive medicine and to a shift in genetics from exploration to engineering. It helps to see all three of these areas as interlinked and inter-influential. It is also important to examine the considerable economic incentives in each of these areas.

The externalization of conception: IVF in humans

The historian K.J. Betteridge provides a careful map of the history of embryo transfer and clearly links reproductive science with the business of meat and dairy production. To begin, Walter Heape, the 19th-century biologist, in 1890 successfully transferred a rabbit embryo from its genetic mother to another rabbit host, where success meant only establishing a pregnancy, not bringing the transferred embryo to term and a live birth. Heape's experimentation was scientific and designed to advance reproductive biology which became a significant driving force in the early 20th century for making animal breeding for food more efficient and more lucrative.

It was not until 1951 when the synchronization of hormones between the embryo donor and the host was better understood that the first transferred mammal, a calf, was born. Prior to this, in the 1920s, sheep semen was mailed to farmers throughout the UK and to mainland Europe and America for artificial insemination (AI – the injection of semen into or near the opening of the uterus) which was already in wide use by livestock breeders in Russia by the 1930s. As international demand for primarily cow and sheep semen rose globally, techniques to freeze, store and transport semen were quickly developed. And there was little hesitation in moving from AI to embryo transfer; this would extend the ability to capture and distribute desired genetic traits to female farm animals without destroying them to access their eggs. By 1949, a Texan farming and research unit had attempted embryo transfer in over 750 cows over seven years anticipating the commercial prospects for controlling and transporting embryos with desired genetic traits in both parents. Because male and female mammalian reproduction differs, it took longer to perfect the techniques required for embryo and egg retrieval, freezing and storage. Rat viability tests at Yale University in 1933 helped develop hormone synchronization between embryo donors and recipients, while cancer research in mice in 1935 helped with embryo transfer techniques. Almost a decade later and just as the Second World War was coming to an end, cow embryos were produced using hyperovulation: artificially increasing hormones to stimulate ovulation or the ripening of eggs in the ovary so that more than the usual number of eggs mature at once. In 1951, a group of University of Edinburgh scientists started using embryo transfer in mice during their research into the new territory of the double helix and gene-carrying DNA. One of these genetic scientists was Robert Edwards commonly considered "the father" of IVF.

Edwards was not the only one interested in medically applying reproductive theory developed since the early 20th century. The popular historian of medicine Robin Marantz Henig provides a detailed account of the New York-based physician Landrum Shettles and his early 1970s clumsy attempts at IVF years before Edwards announced his success in 1979. However, as his biographer Martin Johnson explains, Edward's story is the best known and is also an important example of how IVF merged the once separated activities involved in genetic science and reproductive medicine. The human gene had been described mid-century, the Western world was picking itself up after the Second World War and Edwards was exploring, chiefly in mice, genetic pathologies or how things can go wrong genetically at the point of conception. He believed there was a relationship between egg maturation and genetic formation; any problem in the process of egg maturation, especially with the "chromosomal dance," could become a genetic problem. This is why Edwards eventually worked with the ovulatory hormone human chorionic gonadotrophin or hCG: he wanted to try and replicate the internal process of egg maturation outside the body so he could study it. He succeeded, as had the reproductive contraceptive developers Pincus (in the 1930s) and Min-Chueh Chang (in the 1950s) with rabbit and human eggs, respectively.

As you learn more about how to prevent conception, so you learn more about how to activate it; they are two points on opposite ends of the same axis or seesaw. In 1963, Edwards moved his research to Cambridge University and continued to work on hyperovulation in a climate much more favourable in contraception than in conception. His work there throughout the 1960s was funded by the US Ford Foundation, which was looking for ways to implement world population control policies. In the 1970s, Edwards continued to work on hyperovulation protocols with his wife, the scientist Ruth Fowler. Edwards' Cambridge University research group expanded their work to examine the hormonal influences on follicle development and early pregnancy. His biographer, Johnson, maintains that throughout this time, Edwards was keen to succeed with IVF in humans. Although human eggs may have been hyperovulated before, none had been fertilized, implanted and brought to term – as had been the case with rabbits, hamsters and cows – largely due to the difficulty in getting access to human eggs, especially in the UK. It was this barrier that led Edwards to the US to work with the fertility specialist couple, Georgeanna Jones (a reproductive endocrinologist) and Howard Jones (a gynaecological surgeon and infertility specialist), for six weeks in 1965. Because of their gynaecological practice, the Jones had regular access to human eggs. They were pleased to allow young Edwards the chance to confirm his egg maturation findings in human reproductive tissue.

The next hurdle was to prepare or capacitate the sperm for external or *in vitro* fertilization of matured eggs, which Edwards and his team managed to do three years later. Now the problem was clinical: they needed a woman to impregnate. And they needed a valid reason to do so.

According to the Embryo Project at Monash University in Melbourne, Australia, the gynaecologist Carl Wood achieved one of the world's first IVF pregnancies in 1973 and the first full-term IVF pregnancy from a frozen embryo in 1980. The Jones were also instrumental in developing IVF techniques and fostering the medically assisted conception in the US. And before the two Jones, Shettles and Wood, there was Miriam Menkin, who may have been the first to succeed in externally fertilizing human gametes. Menkin, although medically trained, ended up as a lab technician working for the US obstetrician and gynaecologist John Rock, who, besides being instrumental in developing the contraceptive Pill, was working at the same time on infertility, the other end of the seesaw. Menkin's job was to expose human eggs to human sperm in a glass (Petri) dish to see if a fertilized egg would result. The science journalist Rachel Gross reports that in 1944, Menkin forgot to time the exposure, which was meant to be limited to 30 minutes, and left the human gametes together for over an hour. The cells fused and the eggs started to divide.

Johnson describes Edwards as "a man of extraordinary energy and drive," while Henig describes him as "one of the youngest of the IVF mafia don." And it was this drive and competition among the reproductive mafia that ultimately led to Edwards striking up a partnership in his home country with the gynaecologist Patrick Steptoe; the birth of Louise Joy Brown gave them widespread and almost folkloric recognition as the fathers of IVF. Edwards also played a central role in the establishment of the European Society of Human Reproduction and Embryology (ESHRE) and in the creation of one of the world's first stand-alone IVF clinics, Bourn Hall. And it was Edwards who was awarded the Nobel Prize in 2010 for the development of IVF in humans.

Once the world heard about the first "test-tube baby," the floodgates opened. Edwards and his clinical partner Steptoe established the private fertility clinic at Bourn Hall near Cambridge in 1980. About the same time, the two Jones established the first US IVF clinic at the Virginia Medical School, Norfolk, Virginia. At Monash University in Melbourne a very successful early IVF practice was established in 1984 by Wood. Between these three key sites in IVF's early development, a robust competition emerged: the first American IVF baby was born at the Jones' clinic in May 1981 but with very few to follow in the years immediately following. The embryologist Alan Trounson was among the first worldwide to encourage and develop early hormone protocols for hyperovulation in IVF practice. This explained the Australians' early success in establishing IVF pregnancies. Initially, hyperovulation was a lab technique used in mice to generate as much research material as possible and a technique used in animal husbandry to create as many valuable embryos for implantation as possible. It would quickly become commonplace in medical practice.

Despite Edward's success in the lab with hyperovulation during the late 1970s and early 1980s, it was not used initially in IVF practice in the UK, including in the birth of Louise Brown. Multiple eggs meant more embryos, allowing for multiple implantations at one time, and a higher implantation rate. As a result, the initial rates for establishing a pregnancy, for take-home babies and for multiple births were higher in Australia than in the first clinics in the UK and the US. Very quickly, hyperovulation became the norm in IVF practice, as the number of gynaecological clinics offering IVF and related services, as well as stand-alone infertility clinics, began to multiply; ten years after the birth of Louise Brown, there were over 50 clinics practising IVF in the UK alone. The reason for human IVF was now clearly established: assisted conception.

Before the birth of the first test-tube baby, the state of modern infertility medicine was spotty to say the least. Advances in the knowledge of reproductive hormones since the early part of the 20th century allowed for a fairly crude application of drugs derived from female reproductive hormones responsible for the ripening and release of human eggs from the ovary: hCG. Harvard-based Menkin initially worked with Rock's partner Pincus in developing the Pill, and then worked with Rock on distilling hCG extracted from rabbit pituitary glands. Pincus was able to hyperovulate rabbits to create and implant embryos. Applying this knowledge and technique medically led to the development of the drug Clomid (Clomiphene) in the 1950s by the US chemist Frank Palopoli. It was not unusual for obstetricians and gynaecologists to prescribe a treatment with Clomid (commonly known as a fertility drug) in women who had difficulty conceiving (diagnosed when a heterosexual married couple tried for several years with no success at pregnancy). Usually there was little workup for these women in terms of assessing reproductive hormone levels, testing the viability of fallopian tubes and examining the state of the ovaries and the pelvic area in general. Men were rarely tested at all for their fertility, and the tests available were limited to observing with a common microscope how sperm looked and moved and in extraordinary cases seeing if the sperm could fertilize a hamster egg (the hamster test). If exposure of a woman to the hyperovulating fertility drugs resulted in a healthy baby, all was forgotten; usually there was neither careful exploration for the cause nor follow-up on the condition that led to the difficulty in conceiving. Among the first of mother's helpers were the fertility drugs, implanting another man's sperm without the woman's knowledge to discreetly address male infertility and secretly adopting a child from the single mother pressured to give their child up. This left developing a medical indication or rationale for when IVF should be used with little data to back it up: there was a great deal of unknown, untested infertility in both men and women, including environmental factors, which very few were considering at this time.

In the profession of modern medicine, obstetrics and gynaecology sat fairly low on the hierarchy of medical specialties post-Second World War, just above pediatrics and family medicine and far from the very high ranking, emergent specialties of brain and heart surgery. By this time pregnancy and birth had been almost completely medicalized in most developed and developing countries, so although the specialty was densely populated by physicians and support staff, what they were practising was considered mostly routine and mundane, until IVF arrived with its powerful adjunct, genetic engineering.

The public health systems in the UK and Australia did not initially approve IVF on their lists because the technique was seen as highly experimental, expensive and with very poor success rates (0 to 5% chance of taking home a baby after at least three IVF attempts). In the US private healthcare system, the financial concerns were similar: private health insurers were unlikely to pay for an expensive service that did not work (provide a baby to take home). It is not surprising that clinics, in both public and private healthcare systems, did what they could to improve success rates. One way to improve success rates was to play around with the definition of what constituted a success. Initially many clinics measured success in terms of chemical pregnancies signalled by very early hormonal changes in the woman, but which failed to continue or miscarried within five weeks after fertilization. This reporting practice drew critical attention from within the growing profession of fertility experts as illustrated by a 1985 article published in the prestigious medical journal, *Fertility and Sterility*, by Michael Soules, the Director of Reproductive Endocrinology at the University of Washington, titled "The in vitro fertilization pregnancy rate – Let's be honest with one another." "Competition appears to be the root of the problem," states Soules. Clinics advertising over 50% success rates based mostly on chemical pregnancies would draw far more clients than ones reporting that the chances of taking home a baby were zero to 5%. Also, there is a dropout rate at every stage of IVF, and it makes a difference how you calculate that percentage: do you include all women who started the procedure or only those who became clinically pregnant?

Hyperovulation did improve the rate of successful implantation with the placing of multiple days-old embryos into a uterus at the same time instead of just one. But how many embryos were optimal? That took time to determine, with some clinics placing up to ten embryos in a single cycle and then "selectively reducing" embryos when many implanted. The norm today is limited to three to four embryos per implantation. Hyperovulation was also used in procedures similar to IVF, like gamete intrafallopian transfer (GIFT) and zygote intrafallopian transfer (ZIFT), where again, very high success rates were reported. In GIFT, eggs are collected after hyperovulation, and then combined with sperm and immediately injected back into the fallopian tubes (where it is believed that conception normally occurs) in the hope that embryos would result and then implant. ZIFT is basically the same procedure, but the mixed eggs and sperm are left in a growth medium for up to 24 hours before the mixture, not identified embryos, is placed in the fallopian tubes. With both techniques there is no waiting for nor any assessment of the fertilization of the gametes (sperm and eggs). In the early days of assisted conception, remarkably high rates of success were reported with GIFT, but the question of indication enters here. Who is medically eligible for these IVF-related techniques? Many women who were directed to GIFT had unknown causes of infertility, and it may have been the fertility drug effect of hyperovulation that explained the success or that the procedure addressed male infertility by chance.

Edwards claimed he pursued the application of IVF in humans to assist women with blocked or missing fallopian tubes in getting pregnant. That is what IVF does; it circumnavigates the functions of the fallopian tubes by taking the ripened eggs from the ovary, fertilizing them and then placing embryos in the uterus for implantation. Today, as it was in the 1980s, it is generally understood that one-third of the causes of infertility reside with females (primarily with ovulation; tubal factors account for about 15% of female infertility), one-third with males (due chiefly to low sperm count and poor sperm motility) and one-third due to either a combination of male and female factors or are unknown. So, the indication to use IVF both then and now would be low if used only in diagnosed cases of missing or non-functioning fallopian tubes, which accounts for 5% of all infertility. The World Health Organization estimated that globally 10% of women trying to become pregnant without medical assistance for a year cannot, and if the measure is moved to trying for two years, the rate increases by 2.5 times which means that one in four women worldwide cannot get pregnant when they intend to. The US Centers for Disease Control and Prevention estimates based on data from 2015 to 2017 that about 12% of women of reproductive age in the US have experienced impaired fecundity (failure to achieve a pregnancy after one year of unprotected heterosexual sex). So why not try IVF to see if it could help, as it seemed to with fertility drugs and GIFT? Indication for IVF use in women quickly expanded beyond blocked and missing fallopian tubes to include unexplained infertility in men or women. This radically increased the potential number of eligible IVF patients from 5% of the infertile population to at least 60% which includes anyone with unexplained infertility.

Another important factor in the development of IVF as a clinical tool is the use of transvaginal ultrasound. Steptoe was widely considered a pioneer in safely adapting the laparoscope in the mid-1960s for obstetrics and gynaecology, ironically initially used for sterilizing women by cutting the fallopian tubes. Laparoscopy is a minor surgical technique that allows access to the abdomen through several small incisions and has proved invaluable for practising IVF early on in its development and practice. But despite Steptoe's prowess with the technique, it still requires a fully staffed operating room. This was both expensive and difficult to schedule with women's spontaneously ripening eggs. Meanwhile another soft-tissue visualizing technique was lifted from the Second World War military underwater sonar technology and developed for medical applications, initially in cardiology and gastroenterology: ultrasound. By the mid-1970s, ultrasound was capable of scanning internal organs and generating moving pictures that were visually improved with the aid of computers. Ultrasound works best with a fluid contrast medium, and so obstetrics, especially the visualization of the foetus *in utero*, was an ideal candidate for the new technology (the foetus floats in amniotic fluid). As ultrasound was quickly adopted in the routine monitoring of normal pregnancies, early IVF practitioners seized on the technique for assessing and accessing the ripening of eggs in the ovaries. They developed a transvaginal probe to enter the woman's body with a retracted aspiration needle riding piggyback to be extended to extract the ripened eggs once they were located with the probe. This procedure, transvaginal ultrasound, required no operating room, no general anaesthetic and could be performed at fairly short notice in a clinic setting, unlike laparoscopy.

Finally, developments in IVF hormone protocols allowed IVF practitioners to suspend all spontaneous female reproductive hormonal activity and to externally control when egg maturation occurred by adding back the appropriate hormones in sequence, which made the running of clinics far more efficient. Initially naturally occurring reproductive hormone cycles were the norm in IVF (except in Australia where they were among the first to hyperovulate the ovaries). By the 1980s, and thanks to veterinary science and breeding practices, a great deal had been learned about the hormones required to stimulate egg maturation or ripening in mammals and about the cycle or dance of the various hormones involved. The cycle starts within the hypothalamus at the base of the brain. The hypothalamus controls body temperature and the release of hormones required to begin the complex process of egg maturation. It releases pulses of luteinizing hormone-releasing hormone (LHRH) to the pituitary gland where gonadotrophic cells respond by releasing gonadotrophins into the circulatory system, which is why blood and urine testing are such a central component of reproductive medicine, and especially IVF. The cycle can be read in terms of which hormone is present and in what quantity. Also, the health of the cycle can be checked this way, and often is used today to determine women's suitability for IVF. Once the gonadotrophins are in circulation, follicle stimulating hormone (FSH) and luteinizing hormones (LH) are released and reach the ovaries through the blood supply. Eggs mature and then release a hormone of their own: oestradiol. This signals the hypothalamus to slow down its gonadotrophin release, and eventually stop the release of FSH from the pituitary gland. The dropping FSH levels are thought to diminish most of the eggs' fertility, leaving usually one fully mature egg ready for release from the ovary or ovulation. This egg continues to produce oestrogen and triggers an LH surge which became the marker of imminent ovulation in IVF practice. It was also a bane to many early IVF practitioners, especially when relying on laparoscopy for egg retrieval, as it meant the eggs would be released within the next 24–36 hours and they needed to get the woman into surgery quickly. Once eggs are released from their ovarian sacs, it is near impossible to retrieve them; IVF relies on extracting the ripened egg or eggs just before ovulation.

This so-called natural-cycle IVF (relying entirely on a woman's cycle to produce the usual single egg) was quickly dropped in favour of hormone-enhanced cycles. In these early days of IVF, a great deal of experimentation occurred in developing hormonal protocols designed not only to ripen more eggs at one time and improve chances of implantation, but also to know exactly when eggs were ripe before ovulation so they could be extracted before disappearing down the very narrow fallopian tubes and into the uterus unfertilized. Hyper- or superovulation involves externally administered doses of FSH and maintains the exposure of the eggs to FSH longer than normal in order to ripen more than the usual single human egg per cycle. Sometimes women were given human menopausal gonadotrophin (hMG) which contains both FSH and LH to mimic the LH surge and to control the time of ovulation. In early IVF programmes there were fixed and non-fixed hormonal regimes designed to try to match and control ovulation. Fixed regimes were favoured in low-cost units (usually programmes that were part of a hospital department and had a research arm). These regimes were based on a preset plan for the administration of injections and tablets containing various hormones and hormone stimulators and were used without assays or testing of the blood for hormone levels and without ultrasound monitoring of the ovaries for the ripening of egg follicles. Instead, these protocols relied on what had been learned about the female reproductive cycle, especially the timing of hormone release. By contrast, and typically in private clinics, non-fixed regimes relied on monitoring blood and the ripening follicles in the ovaries to prescribe exactly when to administer the various hormones involved in stimulating ovulation and the ovulation of multiple eggs at once, and when to gather the eggs immediately prior to ovulation or release from the ovary. These clinics argued that such precision led to a better quality of egg and more success with implantation.

With the discovery of a higher-level hypothalamic hormonal trigger of ovulation, speculated in 1955 by G.W. Harris, and isolated as LHRH by A.V. Schally in 1971, came the development of an LHRH analogue (a common brand is Buserelin produced by the pharmaceutical Hoechst) which allows for the external suspension of all reproductive hormonal activity. In IVF practice, this meant that all hormonal phases could be administered and controlled externally, which improved the predictability of imminent ovulation. So, women were not booked for egg retrieval according to when their bodies released an LH surge but were booked for the procedure according to when LH was administered. Buserelin was also identified as a treatment for prostate and breast cancers; this analogue, which tells the hypothalamus in the brain to stop signalling reproductive hormonal activity, also lowers the production of testosterone and oestrogen hormones which play roles in the growth of prostate and breast cancers. In IVF, it practically eliminated spontaneous LH surges that ended in missed opportunities to gather eggs in time and made for more efficient clinical practice with precise fixed regimes. Clinics were pleased with these developments that led to the routinization of vaginal ultrasound, and the suspension of all female hormone activity with the required hormones artificially added back. However, the side effects of LHRH analogues were downplayed, which include early onset of menopause and an increased risk of osteoporosis. And initially the use of human-derived hormones led to a spread of a deadly disease: Creutzfeldt–Jacob disease or mad cow disease. Transmission of this deadly disease remains of concern in infertility medicine.

The final component leading to the development of assisted conception as common clinical practice involves pharmaceuticals and what they stood to gain. Soon after the birth of Louise Joy Brown, the pharmaceutical firms Organon and Serono cornered the market on the hormones used to hyperstimulate ovaries to mature more than the typical single egg: follicle stimulating hormone (FSH), human chorionic gonadotrophin (hCG) and luteinizing hormone (LH). Serono (later Ares Serono) was already a major supplier of hCG distilled from the urine of pregnant women, which was used to treat people with pituitary gland failure, chiefly those with dwarfism. IVF and the need for human embryos allowed lateral integration of its market into reproductive medicine. In the mid-1980s, it cost between $250 and $300 to provide hormone stimulation for one cycle of IVF. John Elkington in his 1985 analysis of the "gene factory" estimates the worldwide pharmaceutical sales for reproductive hormones reached $25–$30 million. By 1995, it was predicted that Ares Serono would control 90% of the global infertility market.

Towards the end of the first decade of the use of IVF in human reproduction, fertility clinics had become routinized in large teaching hospitals throughout the UK, the US and Australia and in private clinics spotted throughout the world where Western-style medical care was offered. But very rarely was IVF offered as part of publicly funded healthcare. Eight years after the birth of the world's first test-tube baby, the National Health Service (NHS) in the UK offered IVF and related procedures like GIFT on a trial basis only at one hospital: St Mary's in Manchester. The clinic was soon overwhelmed by requests nationally, and ended up limiting access to local residents, women under 40 with a male partner no older than 50, women with no children including adopted children and those who had a complete fertility workup prior to being considered. Quasi-public clinics were established in large teaching hospitals where some costs were covered by the NHS but patients had to pay a considerable fee largely to cover the cost of hormones (about £3,000.00 per ovulation cycle). And then there were totally private clinics, like Bourn Hall and most clinics in the US, where all costs were covered by the patient (about $20,000 per cycle). In 1988, Serono announced it was buying two prestigious, private IVF clinics in the UK: The London-based Hallam Medical Centre (a favourite among wealthy patients from Arab states) and Bourn Hall in Cambridge.

New access to human genes

In June of 1986, over 650 scientists and doctors met in Brussels in a well-organized and well-funded conference on human reproduction: The Second Meeting of the European Society of Human Reproduction and Embryology (ESHRE). ESHRE, of whom Edwards was a founding member, had been established the year before and included medical practitioners, embryologists (human and non-human), endocrinologists, a variety of support professionals, such as medical and laboratory technicians, and geneticists. This remarkable and innovative combination of scientific and medical professionals is a sign not only of the broad scope of interest in new reproductive technologies and embryo research, but in particular of how genetics and IVF–based reproductive technology have been interrelated from the start. It was interest in genetics that helped drive the application of IVF in humans; Edwards was a geneticist interested in the genetic expression in gametes or reproductive cells (eggs and sperm). And very quickly as IVF medical practice moved to hyperovulation from the so-called natural cycle approach, the potential for working with human genetic material at its earliest and formational stages was recognized. "Spare embryos" was a term quickly picked up in IVF clinics to refer to the embryos not used for reproduction. Patients signed consent forms allowing their spare embryos to be diverted to scientific research, often with the promise that such research would help improve IVF techniques to help other infertile couples. A whole area of law developed to handle this human material. And various types of scientists, initially geneticists and embryologists, had a new, powerful and very promising field to research.

As IVF as medical practice became publicly known, so too did the prospect of embryo research. Fears of Frankenstein babies and embryos in the lab enduring research procedures filled newspapers in the early 1980s. The British Voluntary Licensing Authority that initially controlled IVF in humans and human embryo research used a full-page photo in its 1987 annual report featuring a giant spike (the magnified tip of a pin) with a relatively small, luminous, two-sphered human embryonic cell cluster hovering above it to quell fears of embryonic people being experimented on. This was the "pre-embryo," a term coined by the Director of the British Medical Research Council's Mammalian Development Unit, Anne McLaren. The "primal streak" and "embryonic disk" are other terms used by embryo researchers and in early legislation of IVF and embryo research in the UK to dampen public fear and to open the way to public acceptance of embryo research. The streak and disk refer to the development of the spine and central nervous cord (the source of sensation), and it was argued that before their development, the pre-embryo had no ability to sense pain. Therefore, it was deemed ethical to allow research on such embryos. Typically, the disk and streak do not appear until 14 days after conception, and so 14 days became the standard limit for allowable pre-embryo research. Scientists are now approaching that limit in terms of keeping embryonic cells alive, so this particular ethical question has emerged again, albeit in a changed social context with routinized assisted conception and less fear of genetic engineering.

The promise of genetic cures was also used to open the way to embryo research. By developing markers to identify genetic-based disease in early embryos, it would be possible to control the continuation of such disease by choosing embryos before implantation on the basis of such and thereby avoiding bringing a child with a serious genetic disease into the world. Given the state of genetic engineering in the mid-1980s, there was also the much fainter possibility of repairing such genetic damage in cellular embryos. Relatively common genetic diseases such as multiple sclerosis (MS) were trotted out as possible candidates for the first markers to be used in pre-implantation genetic diagnosis (PGD). Ridding a world of a disease that ends in a very difficult and painful death is offered as a sign of hope and progress. And at about the same time, the possibility of mapping the human genome appeared on the horizon, giving way to a powerful marriage between IVF and genetics and the promise of control of what the Cambridge University anthropologist Sarah Franklin calls "life itself."

There are two basic types of cells in our bodies: sex cells (sperm and eggs) and somatic cells (all the rest). The significant difference between the two is that if you alter sex cells, you alter all progeny or beings that are reproduced from that cell. If you alter somatic cells, you only alter the cells in the being from which the cells were taken (including those in a cellular human embryo). Using genetic engineering in very young embryo cells for medical purposes (screening and controlling for genetically linked disease, for example) was designed initially for somatic gene therapy only. Altering sex cell lines remained, until 2019, a daunting prospect with far-reaching and unpredictable consequences for human genetic lines that geneticists did not want to try on embryos destined to be implanted in uteri for development into a living and breathing human being, and to this day it is largely prohibited. But the genetic engineering of embryonic cells (altering the genetic makeup of spare embryos) for research purposes only was another matter.

PGD was quickly identified as a companion offering to IVF. It differed from genetic diagnoses of foetuses *in utero*, such as amniocentesis (in development since 1959 to confirm foetal health and used successfully with the use of ultrasound in 1972) and chorionic villus sampling (first performed in 1983). Both of these earlier techniques can only be administered once the pregnancy has reached at least 15 weeks (amniocentesis) or 10 weeks (chorionic villus sampling) because of the risk of harming the developing foetus. The amniotic fluid and villi or threads from the placenta surface are removed and tested for chromosomal abnormalities, chiefly Down's syndrome, spina bifida and cystic fibrosis. There remains a considerable risk to the pregnancy in performing these tests – about one in two hundred pregnancies are lost due to the amniocentesis test and 22 out of 100 with the CVS test; this helps explain why amniocentesis became the much more commonly used procedure to genetically check the foetus. The advantage of CVS, risky as it is, is that the genetic disease is discovered sooner and the option of terminating the pregnancy may be easier to consider.

Once days-old embryonic cell clusters were outside the body, identifiable and with the ability to carve off single cells for genetic screening for genetic inheritable disease, the means for screening embryos before implantation and pregnancy was possible. It was hoped that the menu of possible genetic diseases to screen would substantially increase. Lesch Nyhan syndrome, an inherited genetic disease usually found in males (x-linked), was an early candidate for PGD. One of its symptoms is self-mutilating behaviour (those with the disease may chew on their finger tips and lips as their neurological ability to sense pain weakens), and when trotted out as a PGD candidate, made it difficult to argue against developing and using the procedure. Who would not want to control for such a disease? And the advantage of PGD is that the affected embryo would not be implanted, making the question of pregnancy termination moot. Chromosomal anomalies increase substantially once women reach 35 (women are born with all of their eggs and the eggs age along with the woman), so women over 35 seeking to become pregnant are not only likely to have more difficulty than younger women in becoming pregnant and maintaining the pregnancy due to hormonal changes, they are under increased scrutiny for chromosomal anomalies, especially Down's syndrome, due to their ageing eggs. These people become good candidates for a combined PGD and IVF procedure.

At the same time PGD was being developed alongside clinical IVF came the prospect of a new research material: the entire human genome, life itself, contained in a cellular embryo considered spare to medical use. Types of early embryo research included exploring the elusive early stages of human development and determining genetic abnormalities and disease. Patricia Spallone indicated that during the mid-1980s, both academic scientists and scientists from the bioengineering industry perfected the techniques required to detect specific genes and enzymes (chemicals produced by genes) in days-old embryos. Also, important to later developments in stem cell maturation and the development of so-called artificial embryos was the application of cloning and twinning techniques to the human embryo. These techniques involved splitting the cluster of embryonic cells apart, which at such an early stage of development would typically go on dividing as identical replications or clones of each other. These techniques had been developed in the meat and dairy industries to propagate livestock with desirable genetic traits such as high butterfat content in milk and valuable characteristics in certain muscle types for meat. This helps explain why a bioengineering industry was already in place when IVF was first applied in humans, and why a reproductive medical technique was associated with genetic engineering from the start of IVF.

Genentech, a US-based biotechnology company, was formed in 1976 by a venture capitalist (Robert Swanson) and a biochemist (Herbert Boyer) and is considered the first publicly owned biotech company founded by "gene jockeys" described by Nicolas Rasmussen in his 2014 account of the rise of biotech enterprise. Scientists here were the first to artificially produce insulin (1979), were active in patenting molecules found in nature (first in plants and then in mammals), allegedly the first to develop an artificial human growth hormone (1985) and among the first to develop drugs designed to combat the symptoms of genetically linked illnesses including cystic fibrosis, as well as the first pharmaceutical treatment of some forms of MS (2017). Genetech is most noted for its development of chemotherapies (late 1990s to the present). Common to all of these developments is the role played by human genes: Genentech's founders capitalized, literally, on the recombination of DNA or the engineering of bacteria to become factories for making specified genes, including human genes. Between

1980 and 2001, Genentech's shares appreciated by 2,700%; in 2004 the company earned $785 million in profits. In 2009, the mega pharmaceutical firm, Roche, bought Genentech for $47 billion. In 2018, it released antiviral medications for two types of flu, and in the fall of 2020 was at Phase III of a clinical trial of a vaccine for COVID-19.

By the 1980s, the manipulation of reproduction, including genetic engineering for desirable traits in the meat and dairy industries, was well developed; with the advent of IVF medicine, bioindustry now had access to the entire and living human genetic code. Previously, human genes could be extracted from human tissue, including from dead foetuses. With the externalization of human conception through IVF, live human cellular embryos and the force of their developmental capacity were now available for the first time. In the period around the first human application of IVF, the potential for scientific and medical enterprise was quickly recognized. Although the initial promise of screening all embryos before implantation for all genetically linked disease has not been realized, pre-implanted spare embryos opened the way to a large genetic industry in stem cells, and with the advent of CRISPR Cas9 genetic engineering technology, gave hope to radically alter how we approach disease and illness.

About 20 years after the first successful implantation of a human embryo, scientists figured out how to remove stem cells from human embryos and generate embryonic stem cell lines. An embryonic stem cell is a multipurpose or pluripotent cell found in three- to five-day-old embryos. In normal development, stem cells start to specialize after five days into the cells the fully formed being eventually requires. This explains why a very early human embryo looks like a clump of cells and not a human or a homunculus as once believed by reproductive theorists; the cells have not yet differentiated into the over 200 specific cell types that make up the organs, the circulatory system, eyes, hair, bone structure, muscles and so on. Cells that can develop into any specialized cell are very valuable if you can control for their specialization and sustain their continued replication as a cell line. Not only are there medical applications such as the promise of creating pancreatic cells to cure those suffering from diabetes and neurological cells for treating spinal cord injury but also for taking DNA from adult cells to re-programme them to an embryonic, pluripotent state and creating powerful genetic development research models, induced pluripotent stem (iPS) cells, to replace research on humans including drug testing. The Columbia University-based genetic biologist Dieter Egli, who was among those who pioneered human embryonic stem cell line research, is quoted by David Cyranoski in *Nature* as saying that embryonic stem cells "will lead to unprecedented discoveries that will transform life."

Conclusions

The age of new reproductive technologies sprang from the well-developed, commercially motivated manipulation of reproduction in animals feeding the meat and dairy industries. In order to make the transition into medical practice, several barriers had to be surmounted. The first was to sell to a reluctant public the idea of externalizing human conception and to allow for the distribution of human gametes and embryos. This was achieved primarily by selling the prospect of solving the relatively new medical problem of infertility and enhancing this so-called treatment (it actually does little or nothing to treat the root causes of infertility) with the prospect of controlling for horrific genetically linked diseases. Another barrier was the low initial success rates with what was a largely experimental practice. This was approached and by and large dealt with by improving techniques both surgical and pharmaceutical that made the clinical practice more efficient and easier to control. Once practitioners admitted to altering the measurement of success to their, not the patients', advantage, large-scale growth in assisted conception practices followed. Genetic engineering and the promises that accompany it have followed IVF and its adjunct technologies throughout. Despite not meeting the promise of pre-implantation diagnosis, genetic engineering continues to draw considerable speculation and interest and may be on the brink of realizing some of its potential with the advent of CRISPR Cas9 and other developments in genetic manipulation techniques. Meanwhile, pharmaceutical companies hold an impressive stake in assisted conception practice and profit considerably from both the clinics and the sale of required hormones involved in the procedures.

Missing from this scene is any consideration of the effects of IVF on women who undergo exposure to increasingly invasive hormonal protocols, repeated piercing of the vaginal and bladder walls and ovarian surfaces and multiple pregnancies resulting from implantation of several embryos at a time. Then there is the socio-psychological dimension of undergoing a procedure likely to fail; women are often left feeling responsible. Long-term studies of the effects on the health of children born from the procedure indicate raised levels of abnormalities. And quietly and unwittingly, women and men have become important providers of research material to a burgeoning genetic-commercial complex. So, how to control this brave new world of NRTs?

Further reading

Betteridge, Keith.J. 1981. "An Historical Look at Embryo Transfer." *Journal of Reproduction and Fertility* 62: 1–13. DOI: 10.1530/jrf.0.0620001.

Challoner, Jack. 1999. *Baby-Makers: The History of Artificial Conception*. London: Channel Four Books.

Cyranoski, David. 2018. "How Human Embryonic Cells Sparked a Revolution." *Nature* 555: 428–430. Accessed 29 June 2021. https://www.nature.com/articles/d41586-018-03268-4.

Elkington, John. 1985. *The Gene Factory: Inside the Biotechnology Business*. London: Century Publishing.

Franklin, Sarah. 2000. "Life Itself: Global Nature and the Genetic Imaginary." In *Global Nature, Global Culture*, edited by Sarah Franklin, Celia Lury, and Jackie Stacey, 256. London: SAGE.

Gross, Rachel E. 2020. "The female scientist who changed human fertility forever." *BBC–Future*. Accessed 20 July 2020. https://www.bbc.com/future/article/20200103-the-female-scientist-who-changed-human-fertility-forever.

Henig, Robin Marantz. 2004. *Pandora's Baby: How the Fist Test-Tube Babies Sparked the Reproductive Revolution*. New York: Houghton Mifflen Co.

Johnson, Martin H. 2011. "Robert Edwards: The Path to IVF." *Reproductive Biomedicine Online* 23: 245–262.

McLaren, Anne. 1987. Pre Embryos? *Nature* 328 (10). https://www.nature.com/articles/328010d0.

Rasmussen, Nicolas. 2014. *Gene Jockeys: Life Sciences and the Rise of Biotech Enterprise*. Baltimore, MD: Johns Hopkins University Press.

Soules, Michael. 1985. "The In Vitro Fertilization Pregnancy Rate—Let's Be Honest with One Another." *Fertility and Sterility* 43 (4): 511–513. DOI: https://doi-org.proxy.queensu.ca/10.1016/S0015-0282(16)48489-X.

Spallone, Patricia. 1999. "Embryo Research." In *The Encyclopedia of Reproductive Technologies*, edited by Annette Burfoot, 337. Boulder, CO: Westview.

The Pharma Letter. 1995. "Ares-Serono to expand stake in fertility market." Accessed 30 September 2020. https://www.thepharmaletter.com/article/ares-serono-to-expand-stake-in-fertility-market.

World Health Organization. 2020. *Infertility Is a Global Public Health Issue*. World Health Organization. Accessed 18 August. https://www.who.int/reproductivehealth/topics/infertility/perspective/en/.

6

THE REGULATION OF NEW REPRODUCTIVE TECHNOLOGIES AND GENETIC ENGINEERING

Legislating and regulating science and technology is not easy, especially if the matter to be regulated involves microscopic manoeuvres and entities unrecognizable to untrained eyes. Once human eggs, sperm and early embryos were available to manipulation outside of the human body, it was and remains a significant challenge with new reproductive technologies and genetic engineering of human material. Besides regulating exo corporeal (outside of the body) reproduction and genetic replication, there is also the matter of managing kinship as a result of NRTs, especially with gamete and embryo donation as well as with surrogacy where reproduction becomes contractual and unhooked from genetic lineage. With the advent of NRTs in the 1980s, the UK and Australia were among the first not just to legislate the recent developments, but to use the opportunity to legislate a host of reproductive technologies, including older ones such as artificial insemination. And right from the start, NRT regulation included genetic engineering and embryo research while existing reproductive legislation – regarding abortion and contraception chiefly – also had to be taken into account, giving rise to different regulatory frameworks worldwide. The UK led the way for most western European legislators, as well as for Australia and Canada. Unlike, large developed countries including Brazil and the US that have not adopted overarching legislation nor have they created central licensing authorities for NRTs and genetic engineering. In places like this, there is a tendency to let markets determine practice with minimal restrictions.

Forming umbrella legislation for reproductive technologies; new and old

As we saw in the social history of birth, midwives, typically women attendants at birth for at least 2,000 years, held control over the practical aspects of

DOI: 10.4324/9780429467646-7

reproduction, but not over its meaning. This was taken up chiefly by religious authorities, who along with traditional midwives had to give way to the growing profession of medicine as a de facto authority over matters of contraception, abortion, pregnancy and birth. Despite moves globally to legalize contraception, religious belief continues to hold a powerful place in the control of reproduction, especially over abortion and kinship. When IVF arrived externalizing conception, it generated something of a moral and religious panic over the embryo's dignity and safety. And with IVF came the possibility of transferring gametes and early embryos, thus removing family formation from the platform of heterosexual intercourse and also inciting profound risk to the sanctity of marriage. So it is no surprise that when the NRTs arrived, its legislation took the opportunity to reinforce dominant beliefs regarding kinship and embryo rights.

One of the ways that pregnant people have controlled their reproductivity is to become pregnant out of the norm, typically understood as within the legal or religiously sanctioned institution of marriage. Artificial insemination by donor (AID) is one old reproductive technology that allows for this family formation. Of course, technology is not always required in heterosexual relations, but some of those who wanted to become pregnant without the sperm donor being involved as a parent and or who wanted to avoid heterosexual coitus relied on simple methods for transferring the sperm to the uterus. Commonly referred to as the turkey-baster method, this technology required a willing sperm donor, the timing of ovulation (which was known by the mid-20th century) and someone capable of becoming pregnant. Before people took up this do-it-yourself reproductive technology, medical professionals were also practising it, often without the pregnant person's knowledge that the resulting child was not genetically related to their husband. The regulation of NRTs brought the practice of the former, those operating outside of medical authority, under the same umbrella of legislation for newer reproductive technologies under the shared principle of controlled access to reproduction. Often couched in concerns for safety, due to the potential for spreading disease through infected semen, undetected ectopic pregnancies and unrecorded and untrackable genetic links, AID is often included in the widened legislated scope of reproductive medicine.

NRTs, like abortion, raise questions about the legal status of the embryo outside of the human body, and as it or human gametes (eggs and sperm) are transferred between bodies and become subjects of research. In regulating NRTs, although abortion rarely figures, the same type of questions as used in the regulation of abortion figure, including the definition and viability of human being near the time of conception. And, as with abortion, NRT regulation can weaken pregnant peoples' rights by placing them in conflict with new reproductive partners such as contracted parents, as well as with social controls over kinship and the status of the embryo.

The UK model for NRTS and GE worldwide

The UK was the first to hold a government enquiry into new reproductive technologies following the birth of Louise Brown in 1978. The Committee of Inquiry into Human Fertilisation and Embryology was established in 1982 under the chair of Mary Warnock, a philosopher of morality at Oxford University who wrote on existentialism. The Report of the Committee, commonly known as the Warnock Report, was released in 1984 followed by the government publication of a framework for legislation based on the Report in 1987. Three years later, the Human Fertilisation and Embryology Act (HFEA) was passed into law and the interim (Voluntary) Licensing Authority became the Human Fertilisation and Embryology Authority (HFE Authority). The Warnock Report and the legislative model that came from it provided an influential model for the regulation of NRTs worldwide, especially in most developed countries with established Western-style medical systems.

The central principle guiding the regulation of NRTs, according to Warnock, is the question of reproduction as a human right. This question is pursued in the context of a medical condition, infertility, rather than the social condition of kinship or the right to form a family. Throughout the Committee's deliberations, a heterosexual kinship is assumed and protected, but not as a need or a human right in itself, but in terms of people's rights to seek medical assistance in dealing with a health-related problem. The emphasis on infertility as a so-called medical condition brought the matter into the legal-medical domain. Infertility, for those who are normally expected to procreate (initially defined under the HFEA as members of "a stable, heterosexual relationship"), is perceived as a hardship, and the extraordinary measures represented by IVF and its adjunct technologies are deemed worthwhile to alleviate the suffering of those unable to reproduce their own genetic lines.

Warnock considers how her committee deliberated over cases (some actual and some hypothetical) of people deemed unsuitable to parent, and what should a physician do when such people seek reproductive technologies to alleviate their childlessness. An infertile couple who are both blind, but who have carefully thought through what measures must be put in place to properly raise their child, are considered suitable. Warnock points to how, both in the work of the Committee and in resulting legislation, "the good of the child is paramount." Warnock also welcomes physicians as the gatekeepers to access to NRTs, along with the older technologies such as artificial insemination and abortion that are included in the new legislation. Physicians are granted the authority to determine access on both moral and social grounds, such as in a case where a prospective parent has a history of abusing children. In this case, Warnock upholds the physician's right to deny access to the technologies and to the creation of a genetically related family, although, she adds, criminals can reform and may be allowed access as a result.

Non-heterosexual families are not found in this section, but under a discussion of naturalness and Darwinism, or the evolution of biological beings. By refusing to grant reproduction or family formation as a right and indicating that physicians have the right to deny access to technologies that could help people do that, Warnock, and much legal regulation of reproductive technologies today, along with embryo research, leave a great deal of power at doctors' and scientists' discretion. However, Warnock in 2002 revoked her earlier claim that single and lesbian women should not be allowed access to any reproductive technology (including AID) out of potential harm to the child, and states that public fears over non-heterosexual parents "do not constitute a moral imperative to prohibit it." However, she adds, these fertile homosexual people should have to pay for the service. In 1998, the Human Rights Act was passed in the UK which effectively forced the Authority to provide access for non-heterosexuals and single people to reproductive assistance. In 2009, the Act allowed same-sex and unmarried couples to be recognized as legal parents without having to adopt children born from assisted conception techniques. Another significant principle in establishing Britain's act controlling reproduction involves the tracking of human gametes (now more adrift than ever) through a central licensing authority to make sure they are clearly identified in terms of the biological parents. The Human Fertility and Embryology Authority now does this and under the Act also authorizes who and under what conditions can practice-assisted conception and embryo research, how human gametes and embryos are stored and the outcomes of the medical treatments (success rates).

Another key principle considered by the Warnock Committee and involved in most legislation of NRTs globally is the status of embryo. As IVF brings days-old human embryos into the light of day and outside their normal place – the uterus of a person – questions about the status of the embryo and the need to protect it emerged. The main difference between the considerable knowledge of human embryonic development and pregnancy developed over the last century and a live early embryo outside the human body is that with the latter there is now a much more readily available research subject that was quickly recognized by well-established scientific and medical professions as valuable to their pursuits. Public attention, as well as that of regulators, immediately focused on the embryo as out-of-its-element and at risk of wanton and potentially monstrous manipulation. The 1985 UK Interim (Voluntary) Licensing Authority over NRTs and embryo research featured a full-page photo of a highly magnified human embryo cell cluster next to the looming aspect of the tip of a pin in one of its early annual reports to quell public concerns that tiny recognizable human beings were involved in embryo research. Meanwhile, public and popular media accounts of IVF and embryo research raised fears of monstrous outcomes (cloning, and mixing human with nonhuman gametes), trafficking of human embryos and the artificial management of human reproductivity, including bringing in genetic lines from outside recognized marriages.

Warnock asked the following question: What is the moral status of the embryo? to which both women and embryo researchers shuddered. The sociologist Lorna Weir calls this a matter of biopolitics where, "the threshold of the living subject" shifts from the perinatal (around the time of birth) to around the time of conception. Many recognized how increased legal protections for the early embryo could contribute to increasing obstacles to abortion based, especially in the US, on embryo viability arguments that effectively reduced the window of opportunity in a pregnancy when an abortion would be allowed. If the rights of newly gestated embryos were protected, how could you defend abortion? Meanwhile, scientists eager to work with a complete and replicating human genetic code worried they would be denied legal access on moral grounds to a powerful research material that held great promise for the development of genetic knowledge with significant medical applications such as genetically targeted chemo treatment, the cure for inherited disease including cystic fibrosis and cycle cell disease and the reversal of degenerative disease such as diabetes.

In the UK legislation, a 14-day-old embryo research limit was established to address the growing moral concerns over using live human embryos for scientific experimentation. Embryo research was allowed on so-called "spare embryos" (leftovers from fertility procedures) up until the embryos were 14-days-old, which is when the primitive streak first appears. The primitive streak signals one of the earliest signs of the developing central nervous system and when sensation may be present. As Warnock rightly indicates, this was a position adopted initially only in the UK; many places elsewhere do not recognize this timing as significant to the regulation of embryo research probably because initially there was no need. Newly gestated embryo cell clusters did not survive for much more than five days outside of the body, unless frozen. The HFEA also prohibits the creation of human embryos for research, the implantation of embryos or gametes on which research has been performed and the creation of admixed embryos (combined human and nonhuman gametes and sex line cells) unless specifically approved and only for research.

The UK legislation also brought in abortion to their HFEA, confirming previous legislation's requirement for medical authorization on the basis of health or social risk to the potential parent and family, and this law provides one of the longest windows of availability worldwide: 24 weeks. The influential and early British legislation of NRTs, although initially restricted to heterosexual couples, was able to distinguish interests of potential families from those of researchers and did not use the scientific possibility to externalize conception from the body to support moral arguments used in anti-abortion campaigns. This model also increased legislative oversight of reproductive activity, such as artificial insemination, and established medicine as an authority over such matters. As this regulatory model was adopted and adapted variously throughout the world, it restricted reproduction and increased its medicalization. The UK Act also represents significant reach in the state control of scientific exploration and medical application in a new microbiological terrain that is difficult to police.

In the same year that the Warnock Committee was established in the UK (1982) to address state control of NRTs, The Committee to Consider the Social, Ethical and Legal Issues Arising from In Vitro Fertilization was established in

Australia's second largest state, Victoria. Louis Waller, a professor of law, chaired the Committee and, reflecting the competition between the UK and Australia in developing IVF, declared Victoria as the first legislative body worldwide to regulate IVF and embryo research with the Victoria Infertility (Medical Procedures) Act, 1984. The significant difference between these two leaders in the regulation of NRTs, the UK and Australia, reflects their different forms of government. The UK is a unitary state with a single parliament, whereas Australia, Like Canada, is a federation of states with both national and state parliaments. The UK's regulation of NRTs is national, whereas the development of regulations in Australia has chiefly been state by state, with Victoria being the first to create law. There is national Australian legislation impacting surrogacy, and all Australian clinics using NRTs are licensed and monitored through its National Health and Medical Research Council. The medical practice and scientific research involved with NRTs is controlled by individual states. Of the six Australian states, the four most populous states have passed NRT legislation: Victoria (1984), South Australia (1988), Western Australia (1991) and New South Wales (2007).

As with the UK, Victoria initially mandated (1984) that NRTs be available only to married heterosexual couples. The legislation also called for counselling of couples prior to treatment, and that before being accepted into treatment they had to have tried to become pregnant for at least 12 month without success. It allowed what it called "destructive experimentation" on embryos as long as embryos were not created for that purpose. Later, Victoria passed The Infertility Treatment Act 1995, which established a centralized state authority, the Infertility Treatment Authority, to license and monitor medical professionals, counsellors and clinics handling NRTs, as well as research scientists using embryos. Initially South Australia banned embryo research outright along with Western Australia, but both states expanded access to unwed heterosexual couples living together at least five of the last six years.

Key ethical principles underlying the legislation of NRTs in Australia now are as follows: the welfare of the child born from use of the technologies, an aversion to commercial exploitation of either the couples using the technologies or the children born as a result of using them, providing access to information about genetic parents, maintaining the health and well-being of those accessing the technologies and no discrimination against those seeking to use the technologies based on sexual orientation, marital status, race or religion. Despite this last stated principle, in 2020 the legacy of restricted access remains in Australia. Initially it was common to various state acts that only those medically infertile could access reproductive technologies (including AID) which had long been used by physicians as a valid reason for refusing access to non-heterosexuals who were categorized as "socially infertile." By 2008, as in the UK, human rights provisions sanctioned against such discrimination that has been largely, but not totally, eradicated in Australian NRT legislation and practice. Across Australia, commercial surrogacy and gamete donation are banned and children born from donated gametes and embryos have the right to exchange identifying information with the donors.

Canada, like Australia, has a combination of a national parliament and federated provincial parliaments. Discreet powers are identified as provincial, including health, and all other responsibilities fall under national parliamentary jurisdiction. With NRTs, both jurisdictional levels of legislation come into play with the licensing and tracking of NRT clinics, embryo research and genetic engineering as a federal responsibility, while assisted conception medicine is a provincial matter. In 1989, the Canadian Royal Commission on New Reproductive Technologies was struck and reported four years later in a two volume, 1,275-page report aptly titled, *Proceed with Care*. There are 293 recommendations from the Report including a division of powers between provincial and federal governments. The guiding principles behind the Report include: individual autonomy (the management of social identity and kinship), equality (access to single women), respect for human life and dignity (gametes and embryos), protection of the vulnerable (embryos) and the non-commercialization of reproduction. Both the UK and Australian legislative processes prioritized the health and safety of the child; Canada was one of the first to legislate access to single women and recognized that women have a more involved physical role in reproduction than men.

Pending the crafting and passing of legislation based on *Proceed with Care*, in 1995 Canada put in place an interim moratorium on prohibited practices associated with NRTs including cloning of human embryos, the implantation of embryos used in research, the mixing of human and nonhuman sex line cells, human sex line genetic engineering, the sale of human gametes and embryos, egg donation and paid surrogacy. Legislation was tabled first in 1996 and again in 2003, and eventually passed as the Assisted Human Reproduction Act (AHRA) in 2004. Six years later, the Provence of Quebec succeeded in a Canadian Supreme Court case challenging the Act on the basis that some of its sections fall under provincial legislation of healthcare. In 2012 the AHRA was amended accordingly. This division of legislation of new reproductive technologies and genetic engineering between regional governments responsible for healthcare and federal governments responsible for criminal activity has become a common model and reflects the challenges of governing the new technologies as more than medicine.

In their 2017 study of European legislation of NRTs, Patrick Präg and Melinda Mills note first that, worldwide, over half of all NRT procedures first occurred in Europe, which is "the only continent where legal regulation of ART is widespread." Importantly they point to how not only legislation but also professional guidelines and practice norms as well as medical insurance effectively control the use of NRTs. The professional organization ESHRE (European Society of Human Reproduction and Embryology) has established a European-wide monitoring body: European IVF Monitoring Consortium (EIM). And although NRT use and legislated access vary widely across European countries, the Consortium does allow for a comparative analysis. In the 2017 study, Nordic countries (Denmark, Iceland, Sweden and Norway) were among the top six users of NRTs, with Denmark at the top with over 17,500 IVF cycles per million women; Belgium has the second highest rate at almost 15,000 cycles per million. Eastern European countries (Poland, Montenegro, Macedonia, Albania and so on) tend to be at the lowest end of this scale, with Poland at 2,500 and Moldova at about 1,000 cycles per million. Notable is that Germany, Austria, Ireland, the UK and the Ukraine are clustered around the 2,750 per million mark. A country's relative affluence does not automatically mean that NRTs will be more commonly used. Cost to the patient, lack of information about male-factor infertility, as well as norms, religious belief and laws related to the status of a human embryo help explain these rates of NRT uptake. These factors also influence the kind of NRTs that are available across Europe. For example, in Italy, egg donation is forbidden (but not artificial insemination by donor). In Germany, because of its history with early genetic experiments during the Holocaust, genetic screening and diagnosis had been forbidden since 1990, but in 2011 the German government allowed for limited applications. Pre-implantation genetic diagnosis (PGD) is contentious in all European countries and restricted to the control of inherited disease where allowed. Throughout Europe are legal sanctions against using NRTs for gender preference and for genetically altering embryos designated for implantation. Initially, as with the UK, there were strict limitations of NRTs to married, heterosexual couples by law or through professional discretion throughout most European countries. There has been some movement in European countries to allow access to unmarried, but "stable," heterosexual couples. Single women and members of the LGBTQ2+ community remain outside of legislated access to assisted reproduction in most European countries: 10 of the 22 countries allow access to single women, and seven allow access to lesbians.

The International Federation of Fertility Societies (IFFS) monitors NRT use and regulation worldwide and reports on such once every three years. Referred to as the triennial Surveillance Project, it was initiated in 1998 by key IVF developers: Howard Jones and Jean Cohen. These reports provide a useful overview of global trends in NRT development and rates of application, legislation and policy developments, along with medical insurance coverage. In the 2020 report, we learn the numbers of centres where NRTs are practised by country. Countries where there are relatively high number of centres are Brazil (200), China (400), India (1500), Japan (574), Russia (200) and the US (450). The UK registers only 82 centres and in Australia there are 100. The countries above report among the highest number of centres by nation worldwide, which can be explained by NRT policy and legislation regulating access as well as by variations in services provided and the relative costs to the patient (a different kind of accessibility issue).

Taking this last issue first, within the six countries selected here with high numbers of centres (India with the most worldwide), there is a clear divide between those who offer partial to complete publicly funded coverage (Russia, Japan and China) and those who offer none (the US, India and Brazil). It is assumed that China completely reimburses patients for NRTs, as elsewhere in the Report it is indicated that all 400 of their NRT centres are located in public hospitals. In both Brazil and India, all costs are born by the patient (there is neither public nor private health insurance coverage), while in the US some states cover some of the costs and there is private health insurance coverage. Globally, the IFFS reports for this period that 51% of reporting countries have a national health plan covering NRT costs, 23% have regional or state health plans, 27% rely on private health insurance and 18% have a combination of public and private insurance coverage. The NRTs most covered, whether by private or public funds, are diagnostic evaluation, fertility medication, IVF and ICSI (the injection of individual sperm into the egg). This leaves the costs associated with surrogacy, gamete donation, cryopreservation and transfer, and genetic screening largely unreimbursed. In their study of the European rate of NRT use compared with cost to the patient, Berg Brigham and colleagues found that for 2009: the higher the public funding of NRTs, the greater the utilization; the greater the demand for publicly funded NRTs, the higher the number of restrictions to access; and the higher the cost to the patient, the greater the rate of cross-border reproduction of the transnational shopping for reproductive services. Cost regulates.

So, how does policy and legislation vary in the six countries singled out above? Internationally 62% of countries where NRTs are practised do not require a "stable or recognized" relationship (heterosexual married couple) to access the technologies. China and Japan do. Russia allows access to stable heterosexual couples and single women only, while India also allows access to single men, chiefly surrogacy. Brazil and some states in the US allow access beyond heterosexual couples to same-sex couples, single men and women, as well as to transgender and intersex people. Here we can begin to appreciate what lies behind a growth in assisted reproduction tourism or cross-border reproduction.

It is common globally for professional policies and oversight to stand in place of legislation for the cryopreservation of gametes and pre-implanted embryos, and for control of the number of embryo transplants per cycle. Often a single successful embryo implantation requires multiple transfers; the numbers have ranged from one per cycle in the early natural IVF cycle as used in the birth of Louise Joy Brown, to up to ten embryos implantations at one time. The higher the number of embryos transferred, the more likely it is that multiple embryos implant. This leads to selected reduction or abortion of some of the implanted embryos; multiples in pregnancy and birth carry greater risks to both the foetus and the mother. In contrast with abortion, the control of numbers of embryo transfers per cycle is regulated only in Russia; in Brazil, Japan and the US it is regulated through professional guidelines, and in countries with relatively very large numbers of NRT clinics, such as India and China, there is no regulation at all.

Finally, the Report indicates almost a third of reporting countries have changed some aspect of NRT legislation in the past three years. This change chiefly involves donated gametes, developments in genetic engineering (and their role in embryo research as well as in pre-implantation genetic screening) and surrogacy. Less common types of regulatory changes, but significant nonetheless, include increased access based on marital status and sexual identity, and increased controls over cross-border reproduction, posthumous reproduction (the use of gametes and embryos for reproduction following the death of the donor or donors) and cloning.

Key regulatory developments since 1990

Surrogacy, not strictly a new reproductive technology, has become a key focus of recent NRT legislation. Surrogacy has long been practised and is mentioned in the *Book of Genesis* when, due to infertility, Sarah turned to her servant Hagar to serve as the biological mother of her husband Abraham's child. This is now characterized as "traditional surrogacy" and has long been arranged among family members and friends as acts of altruism. It was also carried out among slaves as argued by legal scholar Anita Allen who states that, "as a result of the American slave laws, all black mothers were de facto surrogates. Children born to slaves were owned by Master X or Mistress Y and could be sold at any time to another owner." With the advent of IVF and the ability to transfer gametes and embryos, surrogacy no longer needs to involve a genetic connection between the so-called surrogate mother and the resulting child; the child can be genetically related to both of its contracting heterosexual parents. And with developments in genetic transfer technologies, this could soon extend to same-sex and trans contracting parents. Since modern surrogacy met with NRTs, its regulation has chiefly focused on determining the rights to parenthood and the potential commercial exploitation of children and to a lesser degree to the exploitation of women who carry these children for others. In the 1980s, in countries where there has been firm regulation of all aspects of NRTs, the tendency was to initially prohibit commercial surrogacy and to provide the legal means to recognize the rights of the commissioning (heterosexual and often married) parents, a new form of adoption. In early modern surrogacy arrangements, the surrogate mother was typically genetically related to the foetus she carried. This was largely due to initial difficulties in freezing and storing eggs. In such cases, in the US, for example through case law, the surrogate mother's parenting rights were effectively transferred to the commissioning parents. Since then, with success in egg cryopreservation it has become the norm, especially in non-altruistic surrogate cases, to use an egg donor different from the gestational carrier, as surrogate mothers are now called. With pressure from the LGBTQ2+ community to recognize their family rights (the legitimation of gay marriage and adoption, for example), there have been legislative moves in many developed countries to open access to surrogacy for the purpose of family formation among single women, single men and members from the LGBTQ2+ community. Surrogacy forms a key part of this queering of the genetically linked, heterosexual nuclear family norm.

Initially modern surrogacy associated with NRTs was regulated to mimic dominant family forms that included married, heterosexual parents, often characterized as "stable." Given the relatively high costs associated even with so-called altruistic surrogacy where the woman bearing the child receives reimbursements for costs, this stability also implies financial stability. But things can go awry in surrogacy arrangements, and they did from the start, perhaps most famously with the 1987 Baby M case in the US. In this case, the mother carrying Baby M, genetically related to the child, decided she wanted to maintain her parental rights and entered into conflict with the commissioning and also biological father of the child who argued that the surrogacy contract overrode any maternity rights she claimed. Since then, there have been cases including whether or not to engage a surrogate to bring frozen embryos to term to inherit property, or to satisfy the desire of a spouse to reproduce after the death of or divorce from the other genetic parent. There have been challenges by commissioning parents for authority over pregnancies in mothers bearing children for others where the commissioners routinely insist on dietary, employment and sexual activity restrictions, as well as enforced medical attention.

In an extreme case in the US, a commissioning parent seeking to selectively reduce the number of the three foetuses in a surrogate's pregnancy to save on medical and child-rearing costs, sued and won that right. In the 2015 Cook v Harding case, the California Children's Court ruled to deny any parental rights to the woman bearing the foetuses and awarded the commissioning person all parental rights including authority over the status of the pregnancy and determining care for all children born from the pregnancy, including putting the children up for adoption. The woman bearing the foetuses offered to parent some or all of the children born from the pregnancy. Clearly this is not only a matter of reproductive technology and engages with family law and the rights to parent. Much of NRT legislation concedes these matters of human rights (the right to reproduce) and family law to other jurisdictions and adapts their provisions and restrictions accordingly (such as the UK Act) which was forced by a human rights ruling to allow NRT access to single men and women. In places where there is little, no or spotty legislation of surrogacy within NRT regulation, the courts are left to decide, or people try to circumnavigate regulatory obstacles.

Over the past four decades since IVF became medical practice, the increased pressure to allow for commercialization of surrogacy, chiefly stemming from the US where it has been allowed from the start, has spilled over to many countries who initially barred commercialization of gametes or embryos. There is now a market for donated eggs (as there has long been for sperm), and techniques for egg freezing, storage, transportation and implantation have improved. When people seeking to reproduce require surrogacy and are prohibited by law or by cost in their country or region, they seek the service elsewhere, especially clients from developed countries from women in less-developed countries.

Even though many countries legally ban commercial surrogacy outright, it occurs, sometimes where it is illegal. One of the fallibilities of NRT regulation in general is its policing. The same holds true for surrogacy. Three legal and health policy scholars of family law and reproductive technologies, Vanessa Gruben, Alana Cattapan and Angela Cameron, recently edited a collection examining the state of surrogacy in Canada. The Canadian case demonstrates well how legislation weakens in the face of determined individuals and a growing market for surrogacy. As stated earlier, Canada initially banned commercial surrogacy, and it remains the case today. However, there is a good deal of latitude in how much women are reimbursed for their expenses, which range from maternity clothing, medical attention and supplies to food, furniture and lost employment. Legal scholar Erin Nelson describes the Canadian Royal Commission's position on commercial surrogacy as "especially pessimistic and disapproving." This is mirrored in the UK legislation, where commercial surrogacy also remains banned. However, what has happened in the decades following these early regulations seriously weakened these prohibitions. There are two factors: increased pressure to commercialize surrogacy from outside of these jurisdictions (especially from the US and developing countries, but also by surrogates themselves seeking compensation) and the serious problem of monitoring and regulating NRTs, including surrogacy. In Canada, the attempt to provide federal oversite and regulation failed at the Supreme Court challenge by the Province of Quebec. As a result, there is no national registry of who is providing surrogacy and under what provisions. Oversite and regulation of NRTs in general in Canada have evolved into voluntary, professional monitoring. As a result, not only is this a difficult area to police, there is no reliable data from which to form policy for surrogacy.

In places like the UK where there is a national licensing authority over assisted conception practice, surrogacy is monitored, but in Canada commercial surrogacy is banned as in Brazil, Denmark, New Zealand, the UK and most of Australia. Bulgaria, Finland, France, Germany, Italy, Japan, Portugal and Spain prohibit surrogacy altogether. Globally 45% (22) of reporting countries to the IFFS in 2019 said that surrogacy was allowed or permitted, while 16 (36%) said they were unsure. Fourteen of the countries where it is permitted (29%) allow for compensation beyond reimbursement. Notably, as large providers of NRT services in general, China and Russia effectively allow both altruistic and commercial surrogacy. In the IFFS report, it is noted that details of surrogacy in general and for compensation in particular, data are lacking; much commercial surrogacy activity takes place in underground markets, including in places like Germany and Canada.

Just south of the Canadian border, commercial surrogacy is a vibrant business. Many US states do not ban commercial surrogacy (except for Louisiana – where it is criminal, and in Minnesota and Nebraska); it is most popular as a commercial enterprise in California, Nevada and Washington State, and as of February 15, 2021, is legal in all of the New England states. It is currently estimated by a leading "boutique-style agency" in California, West Coast Surrogacy, to cost the commissioning parent(s) $90,000 to $130,000. It can be cheaper in other states but may also be more problematic to arrange in terms of family law. In the new millennium, surrogacy was discovered to be far cheaper outside of developed countries and regions, for example, the cost in India is one-half to one-sixth the cost at a high-end Californian boutique clinic. This remarkable discrepancy contributed to a global trade in reproductive tourism that reached such a pitch that India, deeply involved in the industry, banned commercial surrogacy for foreign intended parents in 2015 and recently passed the 2019 Surrogacy (Regulation) Bill that now allows only altruistic surrogacy for Indian families.

Surrogacy is not the only part of the NRTs that has created a reproductive tourism, but it is a dominant reason. Within western Europe and beyond, patients move between countries in search of greater access to the technologies in terms of cost, sexual and family orientation and the level of embryo and gamete manipulation allowed. In Präg and Mills' 2017 study of cross-border reproductive care in Europe, they found that, firstly, most Europeans travel within Europe for their reproductive services. And secondly, that the flow was predominantly from Italy to Spain and Switzerland, from Germany to the Czech Republic and from the Netherlands and France to Belgium. In an earlier 2008–2009 study, 24,000–30,000 treatment cycles for between 11,000 and 14,000 women were tallied as cross-border reproductive care. The reasons for the travel reflect those above: cost, accessibility restrictions, expectation of better or more timely care, anonymous gamete donation and available egg donation and surrogacy. Restricting such reproductive care travel is, as with most NRTs, difficult to police, especially in the Schengen Agreement countries of Europe where people can move freely without any tracking at the borders. Similarly, along the longest undefended border in the world – between the US and Canada – people also move easily between the countries for reproductive care, including surrogacy, and in both directions despite restrictions, such as the legal prohibition on commercial surrogacy in Canada.

The trade between developed and developing nations has been of particular concern, especially with surrogacy contracts relying on some of the world's poorest women as gestational carriers. At the start of the new millennium, India sought to add commercial surrogacy to a growing slate of medical tourism services; by 2011, about 2,000 babies were born through gestational surrogacy arrangements, with at least half of those children thought to be returning to the UK. The total number of foreign surrogacy babies to leave India is estimated in the tens of thousands. Because commercial surrogacy is prohibited in the UK and elsewhere, people are less likely to report and numbers are difficult to confirm. In 2012, the number of Indian clinics offering surrogacy services was estimated to be at least 600, with the Indian Council for Medical Research predicting that fertility services in India offered to foreigners would be worth $6 billion.

In many government regulations there has been a marked move towards inclusivity of access to NRTs. Initially most government regulations and many professional guidelines limited access to heterosexual couples in recognized relationships. Following court and human rights challenges, these regulations and guidelines have changed markedly, with over 60% of countries taking part in the IFFS 2019 study responding that there was no requirement for a stable or recognized relationship to access the technologies, including Australia, Canada, India, New Zealand, the US and most Latin American and western European countries. Notable exceptions include France, Sweden, Switzerland, almost all of eastern Europe and most Asian countries including China. Russia will allow some NRT access to single women.

Considered experimental by the American Society of Reproductive medicine in 2007, egg freezing was a relative latecomer to new reproductive technologies. Sperm, human and nonhuman, have long been able to be frozen and banked or stored, thawed and used in reproduction without negative outcomes. The first births from frozen human embryos occurred during the 1980s. Notably both of these techniques were already well developed in the meat and dairy industries. Eggs behave differently from sperm and even embryos when frozen. Initially, their cellular structures ruptured and broke down during thawing due to their relatively low surface area compared to their volume, the tendency for ice to form between the cells, destabilization of vital genetic processes during freezing and thawing and a hardening of the egg's shell after freezing, making fertilization more difficult. Although the first birth from a frozen human egg happened in Australia in 1986, vitrification or flash freezing, developed about 2008, made the process easier and more successful in terms of maintaining the reproductive capacity of the egg. By 2000, the British HFEA allowed use of frozen eggs or oocytes for reproduction with a ten-year limit for storage of frozen eggs for reproduction. Sperm and embryos are stored far longer, and in some places without limit: *The Washington Post* announced the birth of Molly Gibson in 2020 from a 27-year-old frozen embryo. There is little in legislation to recognize the effort and exposure to health risk with hyperovulation and even less to protect egg donors' rights.

There is a growing industry in egg freezing marketed towards young professional women. Medically, egg or oocyte cryopreservation is offered to women about to undergo cancer treatments (women hold all of their eggs in their ovaries since birth; radiation and chemotherapy may harm the oocytes), as well as to what reproductive clinics refer to as "age-related fertility decline:" after age 35, women's fertility starts to drop; they have fewer eggs and less reproductive capacity, and pregnancies after this age have a greater chance of chromosomal abnormalities. Egg freezing also forms an important part of IVF treatments involving donor gametes. The sociologist Catherine Walby points out that although there is no nation that allows for trade in human embryos including for research, a trade in human oocytes (eggs) got underway by 2010 with openly commercial markets, especially in the US and Russia, demanding from $4,000 to $50,000 per egg. Unlike with human sperm, which has long been traded, Walby finds there has been relatively little hesitation to assign a cash value to eggs for reproductive donation, fertility preservation and deferral as well as for research. And as indicated above, egg donation has become a routine part of surrogacy arrangements to increase the perceived distance between the gestational surrogate and the embryo she grows and births.

The value of human eggs is increasing. In October 2015, the UK became the first country in the world to approve the transplant of mitochondrial DNA. Most of us know that our cells carry DNA (found in the nucleus of the cell); few realize that there are small energy-producing structures within almost all cells but outside the nucleus, the mitochondria, that carry their own distinct DNA called mitochondrial DNA or mtDNA. When mitochondria do not function properly, serious health issues result including stroke-like attacks, blindness, deafness, neurogenerative disease, muscular dystrophy and death. With the skills developed in transferring components of cells for reproductive processes and genetic research, such as PGS and PGD, and twinning and cloning, it became possible in the early 2010s to transfer the nucleus of a recently fertilized egg (zygote) with disease-linked mitochondria to a zygote whose nucleus has been removed but which had healthy mitochondria. Hence, the DNA of the being created by the intended parents is now surrounded only with the healthy mitochondria of a third person: a mtDNA transfer. They can also do this with human eggs before fertilization as mtDNA passes through the maternal line, effectively replacing the faulty mtDNA with healthy mtDNA from a female donor. Because DNA is involved, the procedure raised public concern over there being three genetic parents. These fears were allayed with arguments that mtDNA contributes only 0.1% of the total genetic makeup of the newborn and is hardly detectable when the donor is a close genetic relative of the recipient. Also, the relatively minor merging of three genetic contributors in a single person is often weighed against the enormous health and life-saving benefits. Some, like the medical bioethicist Francois Baylis, disagree. Not only will mtDNA transfer interfere with the resulting person's ability to trace genetic lineage, it would influence research on migration patterns and demographic histories as the mtDNA would exert a ghost-like diversion from the intended parents' genetic genealogy. Baylis also raises the spectre of using the techniques involved to move beyond therapeutic indications to control for desired genetic outcomes, for example, introducing mtDNA from one lesbian partner so that both have genetic skin in the game. Some call this playing God and reject it on this basis, says Baylis, but she says such a path is likely to be taken due to the weight of expectation in a liberalized world of reproductive options driven by consumerism and a "hubris undaunted by failure." And, with the promise of medical therapy, five years later the procedure is legalized, although practised infrequently, in over 15 countries worldwide including the UK, China, Russia and Canada.

Since the application of IVF in humans, the human embryo and its entire genetic code have been accessible from inception. This fact was quickly recognized and heralded in terms of its potential to control for and eradicate genetic-based illness and disease. The valuable research material and development possibilities offered with a fully formed human genetic code was not overlooked either. The problem was with public fears surrounding research on so-called test-tube babies. In the early days of NRTs and human embryonic research, there was little to no regulation of the genetic engineering involved. Instead, professional associations and government bodies developed voluntary moratoriums and guidelines to control who could access human genetic material and for what purposes – research and medical.

In order to avail public concerns over embryo transfer and research, a distinction was made between early conceptuses destined for reproduction and those spare to that purpose or "spare embryos." These were embryos created outside of the body for reproduction but were spare in terms of either number or quality to that purpose. Because of a quickly established protocol to hyperovulate women before collecting eggs for fertilization, there were often more embryos created than needed for the transfer for reproduction (which settled into a professional norm of transferring three or four at a time). This was especially the case before embryo freezing methods had been perfected for use in human reproduction. There was also a visual check made under the microscope of newly developing human embryos *in vitro* (in glass) for obvious defects. Any irregular or otherwise odd-looking cellular embryos would not be chosen for transfer for gestation but kept aside for research purposes. It has become common practice to have those undergoing IVF to provide informed consent for spare embryos to be used for research purposes.

Again, responding to public concerns for the treatment and fate of early embryos, a time limit was placed on how long in vitro embryos could be researched upon. In 1979, the US Department of Health Education and Welfare published the first report to recommend a 14-day limit to growing human embryos outside of the body, reflecting discussion among researchers, ethicists and theologians about the moral status of an embryo at this stage of development. Five years later, the Warnock Committee in the UK endorsed this limit without being clear about what genetic engineering in human embryos would look like. The 14-day limit was chosen for four reasons: this is when twinning or genetic individuation occurs (when the mother's and father's DNA recombine to form a new code), there is no development of the nervous system until this time (and thus it is presumed there is no feeling), there is a normal substantial loss of embryos within this two-week period, and until implantation in the uterine wall is complete it was thought that the embryo cannot develop beyond this stage. Although this time limit to embryo research was adopted globally either in law or voluntarily through professional agreement, this barrier to *in vitro* embryo development beyond 14 days was surmounted in 2020 and the two-week limit to embryo research was lifted by the International Society for Stem Cell Research in 2021.

Initial voluntary bans on certain kinds of genetic research included the creation of human chimeras (recombining human and nonhuman sex genes or the creation of partial human beings) and the implantation of any genetically modified human embryo for reproduction. Like other places initially considering human genetic engineering of embryos, a Swedish government report that became the Genetic Integrity Act in 2006 recommended against human genetic engineering except in matters of "gene therapy" or genetic-based medicine. It is distinctions like this that opened the way for pre-implantation genetic screening (PGS) and diagnosis (PGD) to be approved in many IVF programmes worldwide as part of reproductive medicine.

PGS is the screening of pre-implanted embryos whose biological parents are considered genetically normal. The embryos are screened for unusual numbers of chromosomes; people with Down's syndrome carry an extra chromosome.

This process acts like current screenings, amniocentesis and chorionic sampling during various stages of pregnancy, except that with PGS there is no pregnancy to terminate: the affected embryos are not implanted. PGD is used when one or both genetic parents have a known single-gene disorder (such as cystic fibrosis and muscular dystrophy). The embryos are tested for these specific traits and only those unaffected are chosen for implantation. There is also currently a move to use some of these screenings, particularly for genetic disorders due to structural or numerical chromosomal anomalies, to hopefully improve implantation rates and reduce spontaneous miscarriages with IVF and to add value to IVF with screening against disorders such as Down's syndrome pre-implantation. Currently, about three quarters of countries where fertility medicine is practised expressly allow for PGS and PGD to control against the reproduction of diseases such as cystic fibrosis as well as Down's syndrome, and nowhere is it forbidden. Screening for a donor-matched embryo to become a source of genetic material to treat a diseased child is permitted in 21 countries, but forbidden in 17 others. Although the 2019 global questionnaire of fertility clinics conducted by the IFFS "reflects increased global interest and applications of [PGS and PGD], evidence of improved outcomes is lacking, except in small series and selected cohorts, even with increasingly sophisticated… technology." The powerful promise of PGS and PGD remains such and is widely permitted by legal provisions or professional guidelines.

The regulatory concerns over embryo research quickly extended to embryonic stem cells and sparked an ethical firestorm. In 2001, President George W. Bush banned the use of federal research funds to create and use new stem cell lines and restricted work to existing stem cell lines; however, this ban was lifted by the National Institutes of Health in 2016. German and Italian governments initially banned the use of embryonic stem cells completely. These moves are a response to chiefly moral concerns over the status of the human embryo and the growing influence of religious authorities over science policy and government regulation of NRTs and genetic engineering. Meanwhile in other countries that allowed for stem cell research and development, including Australia, Canada, Singapore, Israel and the US (outside of federally funded labs), a cloning technique called somatic cell transfer was developed with embryonic stem cells, which provided a sort of cellular factory supplying endless amounts of living cells genetically related to the donor that could replace their organs and damaged tissue. It also provided new avenues of research on the power of pluripotent cells and embryonic human development, without disturbing human beings, while "diseases in a dish" allowed for the study of genetic diseases in embryo stem cells derived from those cells screened out for genetic disease by PGD. In 2007, cellular models for thalassemia, Huntington's disease and muscular dystrophy were developed, providing endless cellular research subjects for these diseases. Companies in the UK, the US and Denmark are poised to start clinical programmes to treat Type 1 diabetes or at least reduce reliance on artificial insulin using stem cells; there have been promising early results in the treatment of macular degeneration in elderly people with stem cell therapy. To date, about a dozen cell types, all somatic (non-sexual or neither egg nor sperm cells), have been generated in the lab from embryonic stem cells; great hope is held out for and a good deal of financial speculation is made on sex cell replication in the lab as these are seen as the building blocks of life. Few are speaking of bans.

The business of it all

For all, economics remains a key obstacle in accessing NRTs. In very few places globally are the expensive technologies and services associated with NRTs offered through public healthcare schemes. Those that are, such as in the UK, are very tightly controlled with strict indications or eligibility requirements (including age) and a limited number of IVF cycle attempts (three per person). Options such as embryo and gamete freezing and storage, PGD and ICSI are typically not covered. As Präg and Mills' study of NRT utilization and public funding in western Europe concluded, "countries with the most generous public financing schemes tend to restrict access to covered IVF to a greater degree."

The Harvard business school professor, Debora Spar, analysed the business of IVF in 2006 in her book *The Baby Business* and was surprised to find that it acted like no other. Typically, new businesses, especially those reliant on high tech, start with high-priced products whose cost drops as the market grows and production cheapens. This happened with the laptop computer, the cell phone and so on, but is not so with NRTs. Although the market continues to increase, and technologies such as cryopreservation are routinized and cheapened, the cost continues to rise because the demand is so high and rising. The investment website, Global Market Insights, prices the 2019 global market value for NRTs at slightly higher than $26 billion and expects it to expand between 2020 and 2026 by 4.4%. Another investment website, Grand View Research, speculates demand shall only increase with the WHO report that women's fertility rate has dropped from 5 in 1960 to 2.5 in 2012. Spar recommends that the baby business needs to be moved out of an exchange context (free market) and into a public goods market in order to prevent a classed system of reproduction and genetic health. It remains to be seen what the current pressure of rising infertility will do to public healthcare embracing high-tech conception costs and its adjunct in genetic medicine.

Jamie Metzl, author of the book *Hacking Darwin*, evokes a new age of eugenics, softer in its approach to merge what we know about information and computing with the genetic code. Arguably with the advent of CRISPR Cas9 this code of life itself can be hacked, and currently, this is widely appreciated as a good thing. Genetic-linked diseases, as well as viruses, can be coded which opens up possibilities of reprogramming the code as a cure, as well as tracking the code and its mutations including those in the COVID-19 virus to keep programmed RNA carrier vaccines up to date and fully efficacious. The value of this biopower is literally enormous. The expected sales in Covid vaccines manufactured by

Pfizer, Moderna, Johnson & Johnson and Astra Zeneca in 2021 alone is estimated to be at least $45 billion (and perhaps double that). That is just the vaccine sales and does not include what is to be made from genetic tracking (which has been done from early January 2020) and Covid testing. CRISPR technologies are centrally involved in COVID-19 diagnosis. On the heels of the Chinese-based, and non-sanctioned implantation of CRISPR Cas9 engineered human embryos (what the journal *Nature* reports as "The CRISPR-baby scandal") and in the face of a global viral threat, there is talk of using the gene-editing tool to edit embryos to disable proteins that allow coronaviruses to enter cells (as the scientist He Jiankui announced he had done against the HIV virus in twin girls).

Jennifer Doudna, one of the developers of CRISPR Cas9, and the 2020 Nobel Prize co-recipient with Emmanuelle Charpentier for the work, describes the following:

> To edit the human genome in the way [a biomedical entrepreneur] was suggesting, a clinician would need only techniques that were already well understood by this time: generation of an embryo in vitro…injection of preprogrammed CRISPR molecules to edit the embryo's genome, and implantation of the edited embryo into the mother's uterus… [The entrepreneur was] obsessed with the power and possibilities of CRISPR.

Conclusions

NRTs provided an opportunity for developing legal restrictions on who could reproduce and who is recognized as a parent, regardless whether the so-called new technologies were involved or not. Only because of human rights challenges based on discrimination according to marital status and sexual identity, some of these restrictions were clawed back in some places. The externalization of the embryo has heightened legal attention to its status, and in places where personhood is awarded to the embryo, it has increased legal protection of the embryo, sometimes at the expense of the rights of the pregnant woman. Global flows of reproductive tourism have proved difficult to monitor and legally control and require individual states to react once a potentially damaging flow is determined.

NRTs, their implications for kinship and the new world of genetic engineering they have ushered forth are also complex and very difficult to police. The history of NRT legislation demonstrates how it tends to follow and react to scientific development and technological implementation. Also involved is a now common refrain that the risky business of NRTs and genetic engineering of preimplanted human embryos is worth the promised medical benefits, including acting on infertility, despite little realization of those benefits (the highest success rate for IVF remains about 25%). From initial public shock and horror with the prospect of externalized and transferable human reproductive parts and embryos and test-tube babies, we have now reached a point of social acceptance. IVF is now routinized and available throughout the world and in some places has been made available to members from the LGBTQ2+ communities. All for a relatively high price.

And increased acceptance of NRTs extends to human genetic engineering including the manipulation of embryos to produce children with not two but three genetic contributors. Again, this is accepted in the balancing of risk and benefit. And this is not only a matter of reproduction but also replication. The potency of stem cells has been unleashed, the mysteries of the egg are being unveiled and a global pandemic demands scientific attention that benefits from human genetic science and reproductive engineering.

Further reading

Allen, Anita. 1990. "Surrogacy, Slavery, and the Ownership of Life." *Harvard Journal of Law and Public Policy* 13 (1): 139–149.

Baylis, Francoise. 2013. "The Ethics of Creating Children with Three Genetic Parents." *Reproductive BioMedicine Online* 26: 531–534. DOI: 10.1016/j.rbmo.2013.03.006.

Bock von Wülfingen, Bettina. 2016. "Contested Change: How Germany Came to Allow PGD." *Reproductive Biomedicine & Society Online* 3: 60–67. DOI: 10.1016/j.rbms. 2016.11.002.

Brigham, Karen Berg, Benjamin Cadier, and Karine Chevreul. 2013. "The Diversity of Regulation and Public Financing of IVF in Europe and Its Impact on Utilization." *Human Reproduction* 28 (3): 666–675. DOI: 10.1093/humrep/des418.

CBC News. 2018. "Chinese scientist reports 3rd pregnancy in baby-gene editing experiment." *CBC*. Accessed 3 February 2021. https://www.cbc.ca/news/health/chinese-scientist-proud-gene-edited-babies-1.4923439?fbclid=IwAR3jQVYdr54AweFGU-9CGyvB4o_gJwVqizX8hS4VkNiiaYb-eewdMpusfLIk.

Cyranoski, David. 2019. "The CRISPR-Baby Scandal: What's Next for Human Gene Editing." *Nature*. Accessed 5 May 2021. https://www.nature.com/articles/d41586-019-00673-1.

Doudna, Jennifer A., and Samuel H. Sternberg. 2017. *A Crack in Creation: Gene Editing and the Unthinkable Power to Control Evolution*. New York: Houghton Mifflin Harcourt.

Global Market Insights. 2020. "Assisted reproductive technology market size by procedure." https://www.gminsights.com/industry-analysis/assisted-reproductive-technology-market.

Government of Canada. 1994. *Proceed with Care—Final Report of the Royal Commission on New Reproductive Technologies*. Edited by Political and Social Affairs. Ottawa: Government of Canada.

Government of Canada. 2016. *Assisted Human Reproduction Act*. Edited by Minister of Justice. Ottawa: Government of Canada.

Gruben, Vanessa, Alana Cattapan, and Angela Cameron, eds. 2018. *Surrogacy in Canada: Critical Perspectives in Law and Policy* Toronto: Irwin Law.

Haberman, Clyde. 2014. "Baby M and the question of surrogate motherhood." *The New York Times*. Accessed 1 July 2021. https://www.nytimes.com/2014/03/24/us/baby-m-and-the-question-of-surrogate-motherhood.html.

"International Federation of Fertility Societies' Surveillance (IFFS). 2019: Global Trends in Reproductive Policy and Practice, 8th Edition." *Global Reproductive Health* 4 (1): 1–138. DOI: 10.1097/GRH.0000000000000029.

Lati, Marisa. 2020. "Meet molly, the baby who came from an Embryo Frozen when her mom was a year old." *The Washington Post.* Accessed 22 February 2021. https://www.washingtonpost.com/lifestyle/2020/12/03/embryo-frozen-27-years-ago-live-birth/.

Metzl, Jamie. 2019. *Hacking Darwin: Genetic Engineering and the Future of Humanity.* Naperville, IL: Sourcebooks.

Mueller, Benjamin. 2019. "U.K. backs gay marriage and abortion rights in Irish province." *The New York Times,* July 10.

Nelson, Erin. 2018. "Desperately Seeking Surrogates: Thoughts on Canada's Emergence as an International Surrogacy Destination." In *Surrogacy in Canada: Critical Perspectives in Law and Policy,* edited by Vanessa Gruben, Alana Cattapan, and Angela Cameron, 213–243. Toronto: Irwin Law.

Präg, Patricia, and Melinda Mills. 2017. "Assisted Reproductive Technologies in Europe. Usage and Regulation in the Context of Cross-Border Reproductive Care." In *Childlessness in Europe, Patterns, Causes and Contexts. Demographic Research Monographs,* edited by M. Kreyenfeld and D. Konietzka, 289–309. New York: Springer.

Riezzo, Irene, argherita Neri, Stefania Bello, Cristoforo Pomara, and Emanuela Turillazzi. 2016. "Italian Law on Medically Assisted Reproduction: Do Women's Autonomy and Health Matter?" *BMC Women's Health* 16 (44): 1–7. DOI: 10.1186/s12905-016-0324-4.

Spar, Debora. 2006. *The Baby Business: How Money, Science, and Politics Drive the Commerce of Conception.* Boston, MA: Harvard Business School Press.

Srivastava, Astha. 2021. "The Surrogacy Regulation (2019) Bill of India: A Critique." *Journal of International Women's Studies* 22(1): 139–152. https://vc.bridgew.edu/jiws/vol22/iss1/8.

Waldby, Catherina. 2015. "The Oocyte Market and Social Egg Freezing: From Scarcity to Singularity." *Journal of Cultural Economy* 8 (3): 275–291. DOI: 10.1080/17530350.2015.1039457.

Warnock, Mary. 2002. *Making Babies: Is There a Right to Have Children.* Oxford: Oxford University Press.

Weir, Lorna. 1997. "Australian Legislation on Infertility Treatments." In *Governing Medically Assisted Human Reproduction,* edited by Lorna Weir, 91–95. Toronto: University of Toronto Centre of Criminology.

Weir, Lorna. 2006. *Pregnancy, Risk and Biopolitics: On the Threshold of the Living Subject.* London and New York: Routledge.

West Coast Surrogacy. Accessed 2 February 2021. https://www.westcoastsurrogacy.com.

7

REPRODUCTIVE RIGHTS AND REPRODUCTIVE JUSTICE IN THE FACE OF NRTs

As soon as new reproductive technologies emerged as IVF in the late 1970s, feminists, religious authorities and later gay rights activists responded with different opinions on what was at stake. Some feminists adopted positions on NRTs through a lens focused on women's reproductive rights and health, while most religious groups defended the dignity of the embryo and proper kinship arrangements. LGBTQ2+ activists saw NRTs as a route to addressing their reproductive rights. Since initial responses, feminists and others have broadened issues of concern within a reproductive justice framework that bridges the so-called old and new technologies, reveals the ties between assisted conception and population control within national and global socio-economic disparities, recognizes the queering of kinship, and questions the ethics of replication through genetic engineering.

Initial responses to NRTs

One of the first organized responses to NRTs following the birth of Louise Brown in 1979 was by a group called the Feminist International Network of Resistance to Reproductive and Genetic Engineering (FINRRAGE). A group of women interested in developing issues of reproduction met at the Second International Interdisciplinary Congress of Women in the Netherlands in 1984 and formed the Feminist International Network on New Reproductive Technologies (FINRET). The following year the network of women formed the Women's Emergency Conference on the New Reproductive Technologies and 74 women from 20 countries met in Sweden. Here they developed a perspective that NRTs were tightly engaged with genetic engineering and renamed the group to FINRRAGE to reflect this. Their initial list of concerns included emerging

DOI: 10.4324/9780429467646-8

methods of long-acting hormonal implants and injections tied to new strategies of population control among the most vulnerable, the level of experimentation on women involved in the nascent NRTs, the extension of existing sex selection during pregnancy (with fetal ultrasound and abortion) to pre-implantation diagnosis and ecological and economic threats posed by genetic engineering in agriculture.

Among the early members of FINRRAGE were scholars, including scientists, as well as a variety of activists: Renate Duelli Klein, a trained biologist and one of the editors of *Test-Tube Women – What Future for Motherhood* (1984), Patricia Spallone, a research biochemist and author of *Beyond Conception – The New Politics of Reproduction* (1989), and Janice Raymond, a feminist medical ethicist and author of *Women as Wombs – Reproductive Technologies and the Battle Over Women's Freedom* (1993). Activists included Gena Corea, an independent feminist scholar and journalist focused on exposing violence and malpractice against women and the author of *The Mother Machine – Reproductive Technologies from Artificial insemination to Artificial Wombs* (1985), Vandana Shiva, Indian scholar, ecofeminist and author of *Staying Alive – Women, Ecology and Development* (1988), and Farida Akhter, co-founder of the Bangladeshi community-based equity and justice organization UBINIG and publisher of *The Comilla Declaration* (1989) by FINRRAGE .

This networked array of various feminists concerned with NRTs and genetic engineering was global, was quickly engaged with making connections to structural marginalization and was effective in getting critical views published. The feminist sociologist Stevienna de Saille writes a history of FINRAGE, *Knowledge as Resistance* (2017), where she argues that the group provided a "cognitive praxis" in feminist resistance to dominant science and medical trends in reproduction. People associated with FINRRAGE argued that NRTs in general and surrogacy in particular were what the feminist political scientist Somer Brodribb called a "command performance" orchestrated by patriarchal and commercial interests with little regard to the women involved, whereas others saw surrogacy as an opportunity for women to profit, literally, from their reproductive capacities (see the sociologist, Michelle Stanworth's 1987 collection: *Reproductive Technologies: Gender, Motherhood and Medicine*). There were also brief overtures from organized religious groups to join forces with women's groups in opposing NRTs; the crucial distinction being that feminists focused on women's rights and the religious groups valorized maternity under restricted conditions and sought the extension of human rights to the embryo.

Much early criticism of NRTs revisited earlier feminist medicalization analysis including experimentation on women and their foetuses as with thalidomide. With NRTs, the focus was on the hormones used in the hyperstimulation protocols of IVF including the transmission of Creutzfeldt–Jacob disease (CJD – a brain wasting disease commonly known in cows as mad cow disease). Deadly symptoms can emerge decades after exposure and started to appear in women who underwent IVF. A pituitary hormone (hPG or human pituitary gonadotrophin) derived from dead bodies and used in IVF (as well as in children treated with growth hormones) was the culprit discovered in 1992 by the feminist critic of NRTs Klein (also a neurobiologist) and reported by Ian Anderson. Since then, fertility hormones have largely been produced in the lab rather than derived from human sources. However, in 2011, the Canadian national newspaper, *The Globe and Mail*, announced that especially post-menopausal women's urine remained the source for about two-thirds of fertility drugs and that there was a heightened risk for passing on diseases like CJD.

Finally, an update to the medicalization thesis as applied to NRTs would need to include the early and critical connection made between assisted conception, genetic engineering and commercial interests. A biochemist and feminist critic of NRTs, Patricia Spallone and the feminist scholar and reproductive rights activist Deborah Lynn Steinberg edited *Made to Order - The Myth of Reproductive & Genetic Progress* in 1987. The entries in this collection cover a range of topics including the disappearance of women in an increasingly normalized world of assisted conception and the focus on gametes, embryos and surrogates; how NRTs contribute to privileging the interests of developed countries over those "requiring" population control; and the prospects of a new era of eugenics and genetic-based surveillance and bioweaponry.

The entries are critical of reproductive science and medicine as male-dominated and harmful to women rather than any advance in reproductive rights. Also, as with earlier criticisms of the medical-industrial complex, these analyses point to the financial motivations behind NRTs stemming from pharmaceutical companies, a growing business in private fertility clinics and speculation on genetic engineering. This collection appeared less than a decade following the birth of the first IVF baby and raised criticisms among feminists about how to proceed in this world of fast-paced change in reproductive relations.

One of the world's first major organized religions to respond to the NRTs was the Catholic Church. Their position is based on the tightly held belief that life is a gift from God and that man (sic) is entrusted with this gift as a responsibility that includes respecting the value of this gift. It is God, and only God, who determines when a life begins and ends and how.

Despite initially accepting IVF as a way of encouraging reproduction in the family form acceptable to the Catholic Church (married, heterosexual couples), it changed its position in the *Instruction on Respect for Human Life in its Origin and the Dignity of Procreation*, February 22, 1987. Here the Church introduced the notion of "responsible science" and brought into question the infallibility of scientific research and technology. It aligned scientific responsibility with long-held Church doctrine of "human dignity" and the "integrity of the human person," and extended such to the earliest embryonic forms. The Church's teaching stated that "science cannot set its own rules" and called for scientists to adhere to morals and definitions as understood by the Catholic Church, which include the following: Every being is unique; every being is the creation of God; and a human being or person begins at the moment of conception/fertilization and thus an embryo must be treated as a person.

The Catholic Church maintains this position today, while many non–Catholic Christian sects approve of NRTs and their various components including embryo and gamete donation, commercial surrogacy and pre-implantation diagnosis as ways of creating families. These sects' enthusiasm for the technologies is normally tempered by their views on non-heterosexual unions and trans people. If the sect is strongly opposed to such, they would not support using NRTs to allow these people to reproduce.

Reproduction is of particular concern to Jews in general post-Holocaust, and Israel has the highest number of fertility clinics per capita in the world. Following the genocide of 6 million Jews in the first half of the 20th century, and a longer time of global persecution, Jews are strongly pronatalist. Many clinical and technological developments in NRTs now come from Israel where they embrace a wide array of technologies including cloning techniques for the transfer of DNA from one gamete to another pre-implantation. For those who observe traditional Jewish teaching, Halakhah, infertility has long been a source of shame, especially for the wife and less often as a sign of failure of the Jewish male's obligation to procreate. For devout followers, a husband or wife's infertility serves as a reason for divorce (typically, women are more often medically investigated and diagnosed as infertile than men). As a result, NRTs are welcomed, even in more devout sects as assisting a primary role for Jewish families as well as protecting the future of Jewish populations and defending Judaism. There are variances between orthodox and progressive sects as to what family forms are encouraged; more orthodox sects tend to support reproductive interventions only in marital unions they recognize.

Islam is not only a major organized religion, but it also serves as a judicial component of the Muslim world. The medical anthropologist Marcia Inhorn examines two Muslim sects and Islamic law surrounding IVF and gamete donation. She finds that initially in the 1980s, Muslim communities largely accepted NRTs through the dispensation of *fatwa*s (Islamic religious proclamations) as long as there was no third party involved (egg and sperm donors and surrogates). In Islamic law, the donation of human gametes signifies a third person (or more) in the marriage and thus constitutes infidelity, a religious infraction with serious consequences, including death. Since the 1990s, however, there has been a split between Sunni Muslims (who make up about 85% of all Muslims worldwide) and Shi'ite Muslims (found in Iran and parts of Iraq, Lebanon, Bahrain, Syria and Saudi Arabia). Sunni scholars follow scripture (chiefly the Qur'an) in determining Islamic law, while Shi'ite scholars favour individual religious reasoning, which can allow flexibility, especially in accommodating new technologies, including contraception, organ transplant, transgender surgery and NRTs. In Iran (and other parts of the world), Shi'ite Muslims can contract for a temporary marriage between an unmarried Muslim woman and a married or unmarried Muslim man (men can keep concubines) called mut'ah for a designated time and set price. Previously middle-aged and older spinsters and widows relied on such unions for financial support, especially during the Iraq–Iran war that created many widows and other women requiring financial support. A leading ayatollah (religious leader) in Iran in the early 2000s called for mut'ha to be evoked to temporarily allow egg donation, on a case-by case basis as determined by a Shi'ite religious court with all parties present (the IVF doctor, the infertile couple and the donor or donors). The husband in this case would be temporarily married to the egg donor until the pregnancy in his first wife was established. However, sperm and embryo donation would not be permitted as Muslim women are not allowed to marry more than one man at a time and planned single motherhood is not likely to be tolerated.

This Iranian case opens up further Shi'ite considerations of gamete donations with various questions arising, most of which deal with the relationship between children from donated gametes and their social and biological parents. The questions include whether another man can enter the marriage at all (sperm donation) or can wives of infertile men temporarily divorce them and briefly marry the sperm donor. Who does the child inherit from? Is the child from donated gametes related to a social or adopted parent at all (this has implications for potential marriage between them, and for proper behaviour between them, such as veiling)? Other than issues arising from genetic origins, most Muslims embrace NRTs and do not see it as a matter of humans playing God as does the Catholic Church. Unlike the Catholic Church, Islamic law carries more weight among its followers.

There are two waves of reproductive movements among the LGBTQ2+ communities that have influenced reproductive rights. The first wave began alongside the recognition of same-sex unions in the form of human rights-based court challenges. The second wave is much more recent and involves transgender people and their rights to secure formal identification according to their gender identification. Reproductive rights come into play as some nations hold these peoples' reproductive rights ransom for securing recognition for their desired identities.

Before the recognition of non-heterosexual unions, lesbians had been self-managing access to reproduction in a variety of covert ways and there was no public call for reproductive rights. As non-heterosexual marriages gain legal status around the world, so does the pressure for securing reproductive rights for these couples. Initially the UK legislation for NRTs prevented access to non-homosexual partners, but as with other regions and countries, was forced by human rights challenges in the courts to open access to single women and same-sex partners. In 2009, the HFE Act 2008 comes into effect and allows same-sex and unmarried couples to be legal parents without having to adopt. In Canada, the Assisted Human Reproduction Act passed in 2004 allowed access to single women but also brought the grass-roots practices of lesbian and other women's self-insemination under federal control. Meanwhile gay men sought access to surrogacy and also established grass-root practices with lesbian and other reproducing allies who acted as egg donors and surrogates. Although today many assisted reproduction clinics do provide services to the LGB community, the issue of its regulation remains mixed among these communities. Access to technologies, especially safe and reliable gamete collection, storage and transfer, is useful to same-sex couples and impossible to provide outside of medical and lab settings; however, concerns over the policing of sexuality remain. Provision of services to the trans communities is even more problematic.

Reproductive rights and legislated access to NRTs by trans people are tied up with the issue of legal identification of people who change their gender from that recorded at their birth. So-called gender re-designation or re-assignment is experienced by many trans people as a sort of coming home; finally, they feel comfortable within their own skin. This is why the media activist group GLADD (originally the Gay and Lesbian Anti-Defamation League founded in 1985 New York City to address defamatory coverage of AIDS and the LGB community) proposes terms like designated male at birth and gender affirming surgery instead of gender re-assignment or sex-change surgery. It is not surprising then that trans groups have been lobbying governments to formally acknowledge chosen gender in documents including birth certificates, passports and national identity cards. Many countries and regions are willing to do this, but at a large price to trans people's ability to reproduce.

Most of the countries of the Americas have laws concerning gender expression, as does Russia, China, India, South Africa and Australia. However, many require proof of gender-affirming surgery before birth certificates will be changed, which often means sterilization, and some countries including Belgium, the Czech Republic, Finland, the Netherlands, Turkey and Sweden require that the person be permanently sterilized. As the transgender scholar Blas Radi explains, people who wish to express their gender identity as something different than that designated at birth and have it publicly acknowledged run the risk of losing their reproductivity. This bio-sexual policing keeps heterosexual dimensions of gender and reproduction stable; the image of the heavily pregnant obvious man symbolizes the defamation of trans people as aberrations of "nature." Trans reproductive discrimination is also evident in the difficulty trans people have in accessing services required to preserve and support their reproductivity (such as egg and sperm freezing, gamete donations and surrogacy). However, before securing their right to reproduce, many trans people struggle for personal safety (their rates of suicide and sexual assault including by police are far higher than the norm) and for access to safe, effective and respectful medical care. Arkansas voted in 2021 to ban gender-affirming surgery and treatments to transgender youth; many trans people shy away from healthcare out of substantiated fears of rejection and abuse.

Reproductive justice and the NRTs

At the same time as critiques of NRTs developed, a substantial backlash began against abortion rights, chiefly in the US. The decriminalization of abortion shortly following the 1960s sexual revolution with its new grasp on widely available, highly effective contraception remains a significant mile marker in women's reproductive rights in most developed contexts. The road since has not been without significant bumps; for decades, women have had to plead before panels of physicians to access abortion even if legally available. Many women within developed and parts of developed countries remain isolated from access to abortion by particularly racialized poverty and the racialized effects of geopolitics. Women in places where religious authority continues to hold influence over the state have gained the right to abortion only recently such as in Ireland (2018) and Argentina (2020). In the US, for at least the past decade, there has been a steady attack on the 1973 Roe v Wade landmark decision of the US Supreme Court that ruled that access to abortion without excessive government impediments was a woman's constitutional right to liberty of the person.

In April 2021, the policy research Guttmacher Institute, committed to advancing women's reproductive health and rights in the US, describes 2021 as "a defining one in abortion rights history." An increasing evangelical influence in American politics with a strong anti-abortion platform, along with an increase in conservative judges in the Supreme Court (most notably due to the 2020 death of the Supreme Court proabortion Justice Ruth Ginsberg followed by the Republican-backed replacement with the prolife justice Amy Coney Barrett), has placed Roe v Wade at risk. In September 2021 The Court refused to object to the new Texas law banning all abortion as soon as a "heartbeat" can be detected (heart muscle forms and begins to emit an electronic signal at about six weeks).

Perhaps greater than the threat of overturning this constitutional protection for access to abortion at the federal level is the impact of over a decade of laws impeding access to abortion, state by state. States such as Texas, Oklahoma, Montana, Indiana, Arizona, South Carolina and Kentucky have passed numerous restrictions on abortion access by reducing funding to abortion clinics and abortion providers or making it easier for state agencies to close clinics, forcing doctors to provide misinformation about risks to women seeking abortion (including untrue statements that abortions cause cancer and depression) and forcing women to undergo days of state-sanctioned counselling before accessing an abortion. These are known as TRAP laws: the Targeted Regulation of Abortion Providers. The 2021 report for the Guttmacher Institute tallies 549 state-based restrictions, including 165 abortion bans, introduced in 47 states over the first five months of 2021. In May 2021, Texas signed into legislation a ban on abortions over six weeks in the pregnancy when few women know they are pregnant by this time. The law also allows anyone opposed to abortion, no matter where they live or their connection to a patient, to sue an abortion provider or anyone who helps with an abortion including those providing financial support or transportation. Many of these bills are challenged and fail on appeal and in federal courts. But this doesn't matter; their intention is to chill the reproductive rights environment and to ward off people seeking, assisting or providing abortions. This is also described as a chipping away at Roe v Wade without even having to take the matter to the Supreme Court. And that possibility remains due to state-based TRAP laws and bans both of which increase attention not only to foetal personhood but to foetal rights. There is now a majority in the Court who are supporting challenges to Roe v Wade on the basis of such.

Although this attack on abortion rights seems to be freestanding and unrelated to NRTs, there is a link. The externalization of conception and the transfer of human gametes and embryos along with the genetic promise of embryo genetic research provide a unique spotlight on the embryo and contribute to the development of foetal personhood as an *in utero* voyageur, as well as the genetic potential for human being. From the start of NRTs, attention flew to protect the interests of the embryo: they could not be bought or sold, and embryo research was tightly controlled and reserved only to those embryos deemed in excess to or incapable of becoming a person. A whole new area of family law was created to consider the plight of stored embryos when divorce or death of biological parents occurred and to manage kinship with gamete and embryo donation and surrogacy contracts. Initially NRTs were restricted to the reproduction of accepted, heterosexual kinship norms. Many places still ban access to members of the LGBTQ2+ communities. And ironically, abortion (known as selected reduction in IVF practices) is permitted in NRTs to provide a better chance of *in utero* survival in cases of multiple pregnancies. And so a double standard is set: those who can afford (in terms of economic and social capital) access to reproductive rights typically have reproductive choices and relatively easy access to the entire range of reproductive services (conceptive, contraceptive and abortion); those who cannot afford them, do not. This raises the matter of reproductive justice and the interconnecting globalized social structures of inequity that give rise to the difference in reproductive choice.

Since the first world population programmes were launched in India in the 1950s following on the heels of Malthusian arguments of the planet's finite carrying capacity, there was a trend to tie development assistance to demonstrated lower birth rates in the name of global sustainability. Michelle Murphy, the professor of history and women and gender studies, provides an in-depth and critical overview of how national economies became prime indicators of national well-being. Then, Murphy indicates how those in globally dominating positions of economic power carved the world into developed, developing and undeveloped nations, with a formula for development having reproduction at the core. Population control was based on "averted birth" or the investment in preventing "the better-not born." Contraceptive education and technologies fought for by early birth control advocates Sanger and Stopes as part of family planning rights quickly parlayed into cost-benefit analyses of controlled populations. It was estimated that an initial investment in the prevention of a single averted birth was 100 times more effective in raising the per capita gross domestic product (GDP) than investments focused on production. More recently, these principles have been applied to environmental sustainability: decreased birth rates in developing and undeveloped countries will increase economic sustainability for the people who avert birth as well as improve the environmental sustainability for the planet as a whole.

Mass sterilizations in India have continued beyond the 1970s programmes funded by the World Bank, the Swedish International Development Agency and the UN Population Fund. In 2014, the BBC reported how India has now internalized control of reducing birth rates among their poor and ethnically marginalized populations: nearly 4 million women were sterilized between 2013 and 2014. Earlier, during the 1975 State of Emergency in India, 6.2 million poor men were sterilized, 2,000 of whom died from botched surgeries. Sterilization camps continue in India today (mostly tubal ligation in women, as after 1975, men have veered sharply away from forced vasectomies) amidst widespread calls to Prime Minister Modi for strict crackdowns on what Modi himself described in 2019 as a "reckless population explosion," leading to his Population Regulation Bill. And because India has bought the population bomb argument, as the New Zealand-based academic Nayantara Sheoran Appleton argues, many middle-class, educated, urban Indians agree that more population control is needed, not only to address matters of sustainability and standards of living but to address the desperate and deadly humanitarian crisis during the third wave of the COVID-19 pandemic. Sheoran Appleton states that this perception that India's problem is one of overpopulation, which is accepted internally and externally, has everyone "looking away" from the 2021 crisis. "We need to remember that population is not the problem so much as inequality, and looking away, is."

Today population control has morphed into a much more socially acceptable characterization from averted births to what Murphy calls the "phantasma of the Girl." This is a creature of the human rights movement applied both within and abroad and focuses on the spectre of the young girl living in ignorance and without the means and agency to make her own wise decisions about her reproductive path (keep her family size within her means to support them). This is why contemporary development superpowers (the UN for example) turn to the education of girls as the way out of the desperation of poverty and substandards of living, including environmental degradation. It is an effective mechanism to attract funding dollars to the control of not just reproduction but also production in so-called developing and undeveloped countries. The Girl and her reproductive agency are the focus of global financial speculation, or as Murphy puts it, "the human capital approach to liberal feminism." This is not only a matter of gender as the approach effectively replaces the word race with population: "populations" tend to be coloured and controlled, whereas "people" tend to be white and have well-protected, so-called individual rights.

In 1970, the US Congress passed the Family Planning Services and Population Research Act providing $383 million for contraceptive programmes and hospital grants for voluntary sterilization. Five years later, LA-based medical residents were sued for performing tubal ligations (sterilization) on Mexican American women without their reasonable consent. Two decades later with the reform of the welfare act, Bill Clinton's government linked benefits to a limited family size; if you exceeded the limit, you could forfeit your welfare. The rationalization by the government was that people should only have children if they could afford them. President Trump called for the institutionalization of teen mothers so that they could not reproduce further and argued that cutbacks to social assistance would get rid of poverty. Audrey Farley of the *Washington Post* responded just prior to the pandemic, "What [poor] people need instead of cuts [to welfare] and intrusions into their reproductive decisions is access to employment, housing, food, and health care." Other populations in developed countries whose reproductivity has been rendered problematic and in need of restriction (often sterilization) include Indigenous women in Canada, New Zealand and Australia, women addicted to drugs, homeless women, and women engaged in sex work. A new area of concern involves trans people who, in some countries, have to be sterilized to receive official documentation that reflects their gender affirmation.

Access to NRTs is controlled by a range of factors, not all financial and not all as one might expect in terms of racial difference. As an almost throwaway comment in her highly popular 2018 autobiography, *Becoming,* former First Lady of the United States, Michelle Obama, notes that she and her husband, Barack, resorted to IVF when Michelle could not conceive. She says how she was grateful that the costs were covered by her employer at the time. A couple of months into the pandemic, the *Guardian Weekly* published the story of Laura Barton, a young white writer and broadcaster, who found herself travelling to Greece as the pandemic hit for IVF treatment with frozen sperm from a Bermudian mechanical engineering student. She manoeuvred herself and the tank carrying the frozen sperm through lockdown conditions to access the Greek IVF clinic because it was more difficult to get access to IVF as a single woman in her hometown, whereas in Greece, if you have the cash, no questions are asked. Here she waited for the news of implantation following her hyperovulation and the fertilization of her eggs with the sperm from Bermuda. "On the day I get a negative pregnancy test, 717 people die of corona virus in the UK. For a long while, I sit on the edge of my bed and try to balance rationality and sorrow."

Anita Allen, a freelance writer and author of *It was all a Dream – A New Generation Confronts the Broken Promise to Black America,* which was published just as the pandemic hit North America, also considers her reproductivity following a breakup, while family friends prod her about her vanishing years of reproductivity. In a Sunday *New York Times* article she explores freezing her eggs and her race: "Is egg freezing only for white women?" Although a growing trend among young professional women and a work benefit offered by companies including Apple and Facebook, Allen discovers that between 2005 and 2001, a New York City-based study found only 6% of those who choose to freeze their eggs are black; 80% are white. She finds the trappings surrounding the service "whitewashed" and the cost high, starting at around $10,000, which could effectively prohibit access to those who have suffered long-term economic discrimination due their race. She also points to her fear of resonating with racial stereotypes if she chooses single motherhood and discusses the stigma associated with Black women choosing an abortion, choosing to be a single mother, choosing to have multiple children and choosing IVF. Black women's reproductivity is loaded in ways that white women's is not. And Black women are not considered much in the distribution of NRTs, despite the easy time of it that the Obamas' seem to have enjoyed.

These three women, two Black and one white and all with the financial means to access expensive fertility services, have different experiences of them. One woman so desperate to reproduce travels during a global pandemic seeking assistance and feels strange as reports of deaths come in as she tries to conceive – it is a personal story of loss in difficult times. Another woman cannot help but notice that people who look like her are not in the fertility service brochures and when she checks, very few like her can afford or are encouraged to bank their reproductive potential in contrast to white women. While another woman, also Black, casually accesses IVF seemingly without any hindrance, systemic or personal. It is political when reproduction is a matter of rights or a matter of justice. But the distinction is not black and white.

Meanwhile the mundane world of reproductive health, which is typically measured in terms of adequate access to basic medical care during pregnancy, birth and afterwards, as well as access to reproduction information and effective contraception, suffers from widening disparities across the world. A *Lancet* series on maternal health reported by Wendy Graham and others in 2016 finds that, "the gap between the group of countries with the lowest and highest maternal mortality increased from around 100 times to 200 times difference between 1990 and 2013." Suellen Miller and others in the same series characterize this disparity by too much, too soon (such as unnecessary C-sections and episiotomies) at one end of the spectrum, and too little, too late (little or no basic healthcare, lack of proper nutrition, lack of contraceptives and botched abortion) at the other. They note how the disparity is found within developed populations such as in 2010 when Black women in New York City were found to be more likely to die in childbirth than women in Vietnam or North Korea. Willem Ombelet, a gynaecologist and coordinator of ESHRE's Special task Force on Developing Countries and Infertility, points to how infertility care is almost completely unaddressed in developing countries (except for the very wealthy who travel to private clinics in large urban centres in developed countries). And among the 180 million who suffer from infertility worldwide, according to WHO, those exposed to disease and receive little or no treatment, especially sexually transmitted disease, account for the majority of the infertile – in sub-Saharan Africa, this amounts to 85% of known infertility in women compared to 33% worldwide. Rarely is fertility a part of reproductive healthcare support in developing countries.

So, it is no surprise to find a social penthouse of NRTs with access determined by intersecting dimensions especially of race, socio-economic background, immediate means and geopolitical location. In addition to the contrasting images cast above is reproductive tourism. And nowhere are social justice issues with reproductive tourism more apparent than in the international surrogacy industry. At the start of the new millennium, India sought to add commercial surrogacy to a growing slate of medical tourism services; by 2011, about 2,000 babies were born through gestational surrogacy arrangements, with at least half of those children thought to be returning to the UK. The total number of foreign surrogacy babies to leave India are estimated in the tens of thousands. Because commercial surrogacy is prohibited in the UK and elsewhere, people are less likely to report. In 2012, the number of Indian clinics offering surrogacy services was estimated to be at least 600, with the Indian Council for Medical Research predicting that fertility services in India offered to foreigners would be worth $6 billion. The comparative costs explain India's popularity as a medical tourism destination for commercial surrogacy. The average charge for fertilization, gestation and birth in India in 2015 was $20,000–45,000 compared to $60,000–100,000 in the US. Foreign surrogacy arrangements were banned in India in 2015, although a year later an investigative journalist from *The Guardian*, Julie Bindel, discovered that commercial surrogacy in India for foreigners could still be had, including for same-sex families and single people (also banned by the Indian parliament). Commercial surrogacy remains a legal option to heterosexual Indian couples.

Kalinda Vora and Malathi Iyengar examine the complexities of international commercial surrogacy in India, citing similarities with the US slave trade as both commodified and trafficked bodies globally. The obvious draw for fertility-seeking tourists to India for surrogacy is the markedly lower cost but a high standard of medical care. There are enormous socio-economic disparities within India that create both healthcare services on a par with developed countries and a labour pool of low-paid egg and sperm donors and gestational surrogates. Their low wages represent comparably high incomes for them, and their financial desperation makes for a strong motivator to enter the industry. Vora and Iyengar also identify a reproductive flow of citizenship value from poor Indian surrogates with low social citizenship and protections in their own country to the North Westerners whose citizenship is reinforced and literally increased by the contractual arrangement. They argue that banning commercial surrogacy to foreigners in India does not improve the socio-economic and relatively low-valued social citizenship of the women who served as surrogates. And although the ban may seem to stop the exploitation of these people, we know the practices continue and pushing them underground is likely to increase the exploitation of this already very vulnerable group. And nothing is done to address the privilege behind the source of the exploitation, with many baffled by the prospect of international regulation of medical tourism.

Laura Mamo, who initially celebrated how lesbians hijack NRTs, particularly IVF and sperm donation to reproduce queered family forms, updated her analysis in 2015 in the *Journal of Family Issues* with Eli Alston-Stepnitz to include gay men, gender queer and transgender people, and reproductive justice. Here they argue that by participating in the new world of NRTs, marginalized people from these communities reproduce not only people but also exploitative marketplaces as they realize their reproductive rights. On the one hand surrogacy arrangements for gay men allow for alternative family forms. On the other hand, they perpetuate inequalities, especially through surrogacy. It is this complex interplay of rights between marginalized people that comes to light in developed countries where surrogacy costs are either high or commercial surrogacy is forbidden, only to push the exploitation offshore where labour costs are drastically lower or to where gay men can afford up to five surrogates at a time while the surrogates are reimbursed for expenses only, such as in the UK and Canada.

Reproductive justice and biomedicalization

Initial feminist critique based on the medicalization and commercialization of conception was a nascent analysis of the intersecting interests of state, markets and patriarchy. It has now developed into a biomedical analysis that includes medicine, science and business alongside critiques of global capital flows, reproductive tourism and competing claims for human rights. And nowhere is this more apparent than in the work emanating from the University of Cambridge's ReproSoc (Reproductive Sociology Research Group) founded in 2012 and directed by Sarah Franklin who took part in early meetings of FINRRAGE. The range of studies coming out of the group includes NRT use among Middle East Muslims, the anthropology of global IVF, the medicalization of menopause, studies of moral frameworks within commercial surrogacy in the US, India and Russia, the rise of non-traditional pregnancies using NRTs, human germline editing and transnational care, egg donation and cross-border NRTs and the datafication of reproduction. Here we see intersectionality in terms of globalization, socio-religious contexts, sexual identities and capital all bent to the complex analysis of reproduction, kinship and replication.

The COVID-19 pandemic revealed inequalities internationally as well as intranationally. Vaccines were first injected into people in developed countries, especially those with their own capacity for vaccine production, despite promises from pharmaceuticals and the countries controlling them to supply Covax, the international vaccine bank for worldwide, affordable and timely distribution. Arguments by infectious disease experts that in order to beat the pandemic all people throughout the World need to be vaccinated simultaneously, were muted as in the mediocre relief response mounted in the face of India's desperate calls for help as their hospitals were overwhelmed during a third wave in the spring of 2021: oxygen supplies crashed and infection and death rates skyrocketed. While many within developed countries also suffered and lost jobs, livelihoods, their homes, and access to medical care. Migrant workers and others supporting the supply trains in well-stocked countries, such as those in the surrounding areas of Toronto, suffered exponentially higher rates of Covid infection and death due to living and working in crowded and cramped conditions, with politicians dragging their feet on targeting these essential workers for vaccination. It is this systemic fracturing of society by geopolitical location, by citizenship, by job security, by class and by race and ethnicity that underlays reproductive justice. In contrast to nationally protected individualized rights and liberal promises that all should have rights, reproductive justice focuses on interconnected and population-based discriminations that bleed across state borders worldwide. Think about the unexpected drop in birthrates in developed countries during the pandemic. Many thought the lockdowns would increase the birthrate, but job risks, housing and food insecurity, families devastated by sudden deaths due to Covid and the strain of at-home schooling (predominantly affecting women of all socio-economic backgrounds) had people opting for family planning.

What happens if the logic of neo-population control goes genetic? How will what Murphy calls "the infrastructural distribution of life chances" shift as genetic medicine goes mainline and publicly offered on stock exchanges, genetic research requires more basic material and we accept pre-implanted genetic engineering (PGE) which has already been tried by a rogue Chinese scientist and is the next logical step from PGD and PGS. The bioethics professor at Dalhousie University and a key participant in the 2015 International Summit on Human Gene Editing, Francoise Baylis, examines the new kid on the genetic engineering block, CRISPR-Cas9, which may have a lot to do with our next steps in the biomedicalization of human being.

Jennier Doudna and Samuel Sternberg provide a clear description of CRISPR Cas9 and how it was fashioned into a highly effective genetic engineering tool. *Streptococcus thermophilus* (S.T.) is a powerful lactic-acid bacteria often found in the colon and also used worldwide to culture cheese and yogurt – a significant component of the planet's food chain. When S.T. was found to be vulnerable to attack from bacteriophages (or phages which are actually viruses), there was great motivation to find a solution. By exposing the "workhorse" bacteria to some of the phage itself, scientists at Danisco, a large yogurt producer, found that it effectively vaccinated the bacteria against infection. This not only protected a large food source but also revealed that bacteria have clever immune systems, capable of genetic engineering. When the scientists sequenced the bacteria's genes, they kept coming across odd, repeated fragments of DNA. At first, they treated these sequences as annoying but then realized these fragments were the bacteria's way of keeping a genetic record of viruses that had infected them – a crude immune system involving a form of genetic profiling. If the virus attacked, it would be recognized by the bacteria, and a powerful enzyme would be summoned which would cut out the virus from the bacteria's DNA. The repeated segments that identified the dangerous virus were named in 2000 as "clustered regularly interspaced short palindromic repeats" or CRISPR.

Cas9, the enzyme in the bacteria that acts like a pair of scissors and identified in 2005 and worked on by various scientists over the next nine years, was simplified as an effective and easy-to-use genetic engineering cut-and-paste tool in 2012 by the collaborating scientists, Jennifer Doudna (University of California, Berkeley) and Emanuelle Charpentier (Max Planck Institute). CRISPR-Cas9 could now be programmed to target specified segments of DNA by loading the enzyme with the corresponding RNA. Once it locates its match, the enzyme would cut out the matched sequence and replace it with the desired genetic sequence which the enzyme also carried. The implications were staggering. Since the externalization of an entire human genome with the advent of human IVF in the late 1970s, geneticists have been eager to engineer human genes but were prevented by the lack of engineering tools that could work on microscopic yet complex entities. And the risk of getting things wrong gave rise to the 40-year moratorium on implanting any genetically engineered human embryo or gametes (sex cells that when altered affect all progeny), until recently when a Chinese scientist announced late in 2018 that he had used CRISPR Cas9 to genetically alter a selection of pre-implanted embryos to resist the HIV virus, and then implanted them. Twin girls were born as a result. Carl Zimmer of *The New York Times* announced the news with the headline: "Genetically modified people walk among us."

Both the Chinese government and the scientific world reacted in horror and denounced the research. Baylis points to several ethical concerns raised by the Chinese story. First, she points to how voraciously fellow scientists criticized and condemned the scientist for taking this extraordinary step and grilled him on ethical matters such as consent. Baylis' account leaves us wondering whether this reaction masked professional rivalry and that perhaps there were others using CRISPR Cas9 on human embryos and gametes, but less publicly. Implantation of genetically engineered embryos remains largely untried because of the cascading effects which cannot be predetermined or controlled; it is a step too far. On the other hand, somatic gene editing is widely embraced as more and more cures for those with genetic-related disease and illness emerge; genetically engineered chemotherapy is already in practice. Baylis warns that things are moving fast in the realm of pre-implantation embryo genetic engineering and there needs to be an inclusive, broad-based and carefully reasoned plan for a way forward: replication justice? Doudna warns of the same in *A Crack in Creation – Gene Editing and the Unthinkable Power to Control Evolution*. This level of control in a world so divided by various and dominant interests is more than daunting. How would averted births become averted replication? How would geneticists harness reproduction and those who reproduce to their ideals of who and what is replicated? And, as the pandemic has taught us well, these little animals (viruses and genes) don't pay attention to our borders, national or corporeal.

Conclusions

As soon as the NRTs emerged as something medical practice could take up, critical voices spoke of continued issues with the medicalization of reproduction, especially for women. These included the level of experimentation and intervention in female reproductivity that could cause individual harm. Matters of rights to access the technologies and in what role also arose. Reproductivity, especially female reproductivity, was partitioned and placed in a hierarchy reflecting existing structural inequities including class, race and globalization. Critiques moved from liberalized notions of rights to reproductive justice and a much bigger picture came into clear view far beyond the IVF clinic. Contradictions abounded:

some people were worth the effort and resources to reproduce no matter what, while populations of Others remained a source of concern in terms of their birth rates (or right to reproduce at all). Members of communities long denied access to family formation have to participate in the exploitation of maternity. And through it all runs commerce or, as Farida Akhter, one of the founding members of FINRRAGE, argued, relations of reproduction cannot be severed from the relations of production. There are large profits riding on the use of reproductive hormones; on surrogacy contracts here and abroad; and on the gathering, storing and transporting of human gametes and embryos. And there are unimagined profits in harnessing the power of genetics, which is now at hand.

Further reading

Allen, Anita. 1990. "Surrogacy, Slavery, and the Ownership of Life." *Harvard Journal of Law and Public Policy* 13 (1): 139–149.

Baylis, Francoise. 2013. "The Ethics of Creating Children with Three Genetic Parents." *Reproductive BioMedicine Online* 26: 531–534. DOI: 10.1016/j.rbmo.2013.03.006.

Bock von Wülfingen, Bettina. 2016. "Contested Change: How Germany Came to Allow PGD." *Reproductive Biomedicine & Society Online* 3: 60–67. DOI: 10.1016/j.rbms.2016.11.002.

Brigham, Karen Berg, Benjamin Cadier, and KKarine Chevreul. 2013. "The Diversity of Regulation and Public Financing of IVF in Europe and Its Impact on Utilization." *Human Reproduction* 28 (3): 666–675. DOI: 10.1093/humrep/des418.

CBC News. 2018. "Chinese scientist reports 3rd pregnancy in baby-gene editing experiment." *CBC.* Accessed 3 February 2021. https://www.cbc.ca/news/health/chinese-scientist-proud-gene-edited-babies-1.4923439?fbclid=IwAR3jQVYdr54AweFGU9CGyvB4o_gJwVqizX8hS4VkNiiaYb-eewdMpusfLIk.

Cyranoski, David. 2019. "The CRISPR-baby scandal: What's next for human gene editing." *Nature.* Accessed 5 May 2021. https://www.nature.com/articles/d41586-019-00673-1.

Doudna, Jennifer A., and Samuel H. Sternberg. 2017. *A Crack in Creation: Gene Editing and the Unthinkable Power to Control Evolution.* New York: Houghton Mifflin Harcourt.

Global Market Insights. 2020. "Assisted reproductive technology market size by procedure." https://www.gminsights.com/industry-analysis/assisted-reproductive-technology-market

Government of Canada. 1994. *Proceed with Care—Final Report of the Royal Commission on New Reproductive Technologies.* Edited by Political and Social Affairs. Ottawa: Government of Canada.

Government of Canada. 2016. *Assisted Human Reproduction Act.* Edited by Minister of Justice. Ottawa: Government of Canada.

Gruben, Vanessa, Alana Cattapan, and Angela Cameron, eds. 2018. *Surrogacy in Canada: Critical Perspectives in Law and Policy.* Toronto: Irwin Law.

Haberman, Clyde. 2014. "Baby M and the question of surrogate motherhood." *The New York Times.* Accessed 1 July 2021. https://www.nytimes.com/2014/03/24/us/baby-m-and-the-question-of-surrogate-motherhood.html.

"International Federation of Fertility Societies' Surveillance (IFFS). 2019: Global Trends in Reproductive Policy and Practice, 8th Edition." *Global Reproductive Health* 4 (1): 1–138. DOI: 10.1097/GRH.0000000000000029.

Lati, Marisa. 2020. "Meet Molly, the baby who came from an embryo frozen when her mom was a year old." *The Washington Post.* Accessed 22 February 2021. https://www. washingtonpost.com/lifestyle/2020/12/03/embryo-frozen-27-years-ago-live-birth/.

Metzl, Jamie. 2019. *Hacking Darwin: Genetic Engineering and the Future of Humanity.* Naperville, IL: Sourcebooks.

Mueller, Benjamin. 2019. "U.K. backs gay marriage and abortion rights in Irish province." *The New York Times,* 10 July.

Nelson, Erin. 2018. "Desperately Seeking Surrogates: Thoughts on Canada's Emergence as an International Surrogacy Destination." In *Surrogacy in Canada: Critical Perspectives in Law and Policy,* edited by Vanessa Gruben, Alana Cattapan, and Angela Cameron, 213–243. Toronto: Irwin Law.

Präg, Patricia, and Melinda Mills. 2017. "Assisted Reproductive Technologies in Europe. Usage and Regulation in the Context of Cross-Border Reproductive Care." In *Childlessness in Europe, Patterns, Causes and Contexts. Demographic Research Monographs,* edited by M. Kreyenfeld and D. Konietzka, 289–309. New York: Springer.

Riezzo, Irene, Margherita Neri, Stefania Bello, Cristofo Pomara, and Emanuela Turillazzi. 2016. "Italian Law on Medically Assisted Reproduction: Do Women's Autonomy and Health Matter?" *BMC Women's Health* 16 (44): 1–7. DOI: 10.1186/ s12905-016-0324-4.

Spar, Debora. 2006. *The Baby Business: How Money, Science, and Politics Drive the Commerce of Conception.* Boston, MA: Harvard Business School Press.

Srivastava, Astha. 2021. "The Surrogacy Regulation (2019) Bill of India: A Critique." *Journal of International Women's Studies* 22(1): 139–152. https://vc.bridgew.edu/jiws/ vol22/iss1/8.

Waldby, Catherina. 2015. "The Oocyte Market and Social Egg Freezing: From Scarcity to Singularity." *Journal of Cultural Economy* 8 (3): 275–291. DOI: 10.1080/17530350.2015.1039457.

Warnock, Mary. 2002. *Making Babies: Is There a Right to Have Children.* Oxford: Oxford University Press.

Weir, Lorna. 1997. "Australian Legislation on Infertility Treatments." In *Governing Medically Assisted Human Reproduction,* edited by Lorna Weir, 91–95. Toronto: University of Toronto Centre of Criminology.

Weir, Lorna. 2006. *Pregnancy, Risk and Biopolitics: On the Threshold of the Living Subject.* London and New York: Routledge.

West Coast Surrogacy. Accessed 2 February 2021. https://www.westcoastsurrogacy.com.

8

WOMEN AND NEW REPRODUCTIVE TECHNOLOGIES

Kinship and the biomedicalization of life itself

Breaking it down and winding it up: women and NRTs

We started this examination of gender, reproduction and technological development by examining what reproduction has meant as far back as we can trace. We moved from elaborate prehistoric symbols and carvings through the first recorded thoughts about reproduction, through the ups and downs of making sense of this essential and mysterious activity. Body parts were increasingly atomized, mechanized and engineered. And through it all there was woman. Woman whose body swelled and who pushed out babies, and who then nursed those babies' development. Woman portrayed as a divine creator for these live-giving qualities. Woman is different than man in both external and increasingly visualized internal body parts. Woman as inferior to man in the meaning made of reproduction despite the greater obvious involvement; quality trumped quantity as a reflection of growing beliefs in masculine creators in the abstract.

Women: As modern civil societies settled and science soared, reproduction was funnelled into expected, heteronormative family forms with still potent blessings from religious authorities and a new voice added to the chorus: medicine. At times sneaking it and at times grabbing it, the emerging medical authority over reproductive matters took control away from traditional birth attendants, chiefly female midwives, and claimed it as their territory. Pregnancy and birth were treated as illness and in need of medical attention, and so women were hospitalized and medicalized at exponentially higher rates than men. Meanwhile the steady drum of social control of reproduction by moral authorities continued, trying to keep from women what doctors were learning that could control reproduction chiefly in woman's bodies. And women continued to bear the brunt for reproducing outside of expected norms as gametes (eggs and sperm

DOI: 10.4324/9780429467646-9

cells) pay no attention to religious, moral and legal sanctions and as pregnancy ends up in the lap of women.

And as women, people organized the clandestine exchange of contraceptive information, the development of effective contraceptives and access to safe abortion, because if not them, then who? As early proponents of family planning argued, if women were to enjoy the benefits of modern society and improved qualities of life, they had to be able to manage and limit the number of their children. This was also the germ of the key principle behind global policies of population control where once again pregnant bodies often, not always, were the target of attention. Those most influential in the flow of global capital worried about the relatively substandard quality of life in these places, but most of all they worried about the effect of these growing populations on the entire planet, assuming it had a finite carrying capacity. Their ideal future was *Star Trek*: diverse populations well controlled in number, civil, capable of incredible technological development, never hungry or without work and free to explore new worlds and spread their programme for success and well-being. In the popular TV and film series, women looked and behaved a lot like men (except when an exotic sexual other served), and there was rarely a pregnant body to be seen. This was a universe with no apparent struggle over finite resources and reproduction was taken for granted, like the 1960s as idealized through American popular culture of the time.

However, in the actual state of affairs in 1960s America, the connection between birth control and population control was not lost, especially on Black Americans, Indigenous people throughout North America and Australasia and Others globally. Besides massive programmes designed by developed countries to reduce birthrates in developing countries, the control of subpopulations of women in developed nations occurred and continues today through various means, mostly involving financial incentives or disincentives; manifest and latent. The struggle for individual woman's right to choose when to reproduce and how, became a different kind of struggle for women brutally targeted as bearers of the "better-not born." It involved and continues to involve struggles over structured inequities and injustices, often racialized, including access to decent standards of living, to healthcare and employment and to personal and community safety.

And now the word "woman" is under question. Its reproductive determination has become unhinged as those identifying as and appearing to be not women become pregnant and give birth, and because of the demand for a growing workforce of gestational carriers and egg donors (also neither women, nor mothers). In keeping "woman" here, the purpose is not to blindly accept historical parameters of what constitutes a woman, but to acknowledge a pretty long history of the careful patrolling of those parameters.

And: Why such a fuss about such a little word like "and," and one that only connects normally bigger and more important words? Because the nature of that connection matters. The phrase, women *in* reproductive technologies is far different than, women *and* reproductive technologies. The former speak to gender and the medicalization of infertility perhaps or to the ongoing matter of women's access to a long male-dominated medical profession. Both are important issues and part of the phrase with the *and*. But this phrase is more open, and the entities on either side of the little word stand close but independent of each other. It allows more discussion including the struggle for women's independence from the material injustices, inequities and constraints arising from various ideologies of reproduction. It provides space between the two, perhaps too much for some who see gender itself as a technology or others who see NRTs as an opportunity for women's employment or as an answer to infertility. But those discussions are not prohibited by the use of the little word, *and*. Finally, the use of *or* and *as* paints a bleak and dehumanized picture. The important point here is that *and* is a carefully chosen word.

New: By now there should be at least some appreciation for how the so-called *new* reproductive technologies drag along with them old assumptions about who has the right to reproduce and that medical and scientific authorities always act in the best interests of those they administer to. It is true that the externalization of conception from the human body is a significant threshold to profound disruptions of kinship and the genetic engineering of human beings and represents something new. Also, the medicalization thesis concerned with growing commercial interests in healthcare and pharmaceuticals morphs into heightened financial speculation in fertility clinics, in a growing trade in human gametes and reproductive capacities, as well as in many highly promising medical applications of embryo research and stem cell lines. Various businesses have been poking around reproduction for new markets throughout the 20th century: harnessing the powers of reproductive hormones as anti-ageing treatments, increased medicalization of pregnancy and childbirth through the routinization of urine and blood tests and visual scans, genetic screening of *in utero* embryos to help eliminate children born with Down's syndrome and spina bifida, and rising caesarian rates at birth including the possibility of elective C-sections. *New* meant value-added options to the host of reproductive services available to those who can afford them including scanning and diagnosing embryos pre-implantation to avoid the difficult decision to abort if a genetic anomaly is discovered. Now, male infertility can be addressed during IVF by injecting a single sperm into the harvested egg, and gamete and embryo donation and surrogacy open a host of new possibilities for not only the medically infertile but those called socially infertile (non-heterosexuals and singletons). Again, even this disruption of genetic lineage and non-heterosexual family formation is not *new*. Women can choose to reproduce with people outside of condoned relationships and have done so for a long time. With more difficulty and considerable assistance from women, men can and have done so as well. It is the case that the access to genetic-based family formation is very new to trans and non-gender binary folks and is not available to non-heterosexuals everywhere. Also *new* is a markedly increased emphasis on genetic links to children, again in places where and among people who can afford it.

The social control of reproduction also remains. Access to NRTs is far from universal, and places where infertility rates are rampant due to subsistence living and high rates of sexually transmitted disease are the least likely to be offered fertility services. There are very few places on the planet where high-end fertility services (the NRTs with genetic screening) are offered with no cost to the patient. Meanwhile undesirable populations or ones considered problematic because of their poverty, their dependencies, their race and their sexual identity are targets of plans designed to reduce their birthrates, openly, underhandedly or through neglect of root and systemic socio-economic disparities. With the hand-in-hand development of NRTs and genetic engineering, the technologies of birth control may go viral, or eugenic: old ideas of the social control of reproduction meet new means of doing so.

Reproductive: Our understanding of reproductivity has developed substantially from nonsexual pregnancy and birth to theories based on what could be seen outside the body, and then to breaking down reproductive parts and increasing our knowledge of the natural engineering of reproduction with advances in anatomy, neurology, circulation, hormones and finally genetics. But reproduction is not just science, it is also kinship, heavy with meaning and culture, and we work hard to control it morally, defensively, desperately and socially. The story of reproductive technologies includes these systems as well – who has been allowed to reproduce, who is allowed to keep their children, who is allowed to hold on to their meaning of pregnancy and birth and children and who is allowed to choose when they reproduce and under what conditions. It is a complex socio-cultural machinery that has developed over ages and still varies from place to place.

But we also need to acknowledge the difference made in that complexity of reproduction by the externalization of conception and the exposure of a fully formed cluster of human cells to manipulation, and the speed with which the changes have happened. In one generation we have created the ability to transfer human gametes and embryos from one body to the other so that biological parents are not necessarily legal parents who are not necessarily genetic parents. We can freeze and store human gametes and embryos and play around with time, having one twin born twenty years after the other. We are getting good at examining early embryonic clusters of cells and can now operate on the chromosome itself by moving DNA more and more precisely in and out of the chain. Much of these techniques are thanks to previous applications in breeding nonhuman mammals for the food industry and to a lesser degree trying to save animals facing extinction.

This leads us to the question of when does reproduction become replication. During the pandemic, birthrates in developed countries dropped adding to an already downward trend and causing considerable concern (many were expecting an increased birthrate). The global birthrate is often evoked in terms of environmental sustainability, whereas national ones tend to be discussed in terms of financial sustainability. And in the complex algorithms of national economies, lowering birth rates can reach a tipping point (2.1 children per woman) that spells economic decline: There are not enough people to replace the ones already here, or "who is going to look after me in my old age?" In response and during the pandemic, China recently increased its one-child policy to three children per woman, but young urban people in China hesitate to move beyond one child due to the cost of rearing children. There will likely be more national strategies to address dropping birthrates around the globe as an issue of flows and replication of capital. Breeding doesn't seem like such a strange possibility.

Technologies: The word *technology* is probably the most loaded one in this phrase. It is so easy to reduce it to the mechanism, the specific surgical procedure, the thing. But never is technology only the thing. Systems of knowledge swirl around and through the thing; it does not spring fully formed from the earth, the lab or the factory. How seeds of curiosity are planted and allowed to grow follow power lines such that ideologies (heteronormativity, population control equals development, the medical-genetic industrial complex) are more a reproductive technology and the engineering of genes than IVF and CRISPR-Cas9. Focus only on the later and you see little and understand even less.

What's next? Kinship and biomedicalization in the 21st century

There are several reasons for reviewing the long history of reproductive thought. For one, this demonstrates how ideas have changed over time. For another, it also demonstrates the fallibility of science, even contemporary science. And finally, it demonstrates how political interests not only guide scientific and technological developments, it can blind them, sociologically speaking. Below is a selection of recent socio-technical developments hinging on reproduction as illustration.

In Chapter 1 we saw how even in modern medical science, the human egg is characterized as massive and passive in contrast with the mobile and courageous sperm. This gender discrimination follows a two millennial-long trajectory starting with Aristotle's theory that women provide the dumb matter and men provide the intelligent matrix in human reproduction. Today, the difficult-to-freeze human egg is revealing more mysteries and opening new pathways. In 2021, Nidhl Subbaraman announced in *Nature* that multiple labs are able to generate human blastocysts (about four-day-old embryos) from stem cells. Besides the serious ethical concerns with such research, the achievement relies on developments in early embryology and the technical mastery of manipulating that relatively giant egg as it starts to divide into pluripotent cells immediately following fertilization. Artificial blastocyst generation involves turning stem cells into eggs that are then fertilized by sperm, and this research leads to the comment in another 2021 article from *ScienceDaily*: "Oocytes [eggs] are extremely unique because of their ability to bring forth the over two hundred kinds of highly differentiated cells needed to create an individual person." Eggs are active agents and genetically versatile.

Eggs are a source of incredible hope, reports Sam Anderson, as two northern white rhinos, Najin and Fatu (mother and daughter), face extinction. They are the last two on Earth. Their eggs were carefully collected in 2019 in the hope of fertilizing them with the frozen sperm of one of the last males of the species and implanting the embryos into a southern white rhino surrogate. IVF and the manipulation of gametes, including cloning, have circled back from their origins in animal husbandry to play a significant role in species preservation. This is a good thing, as the UN declared in May 2019 that we face a mass extinction event of 1 million plant and animal species. But it isn't infertility that wiped out these species. It is profound disruptions to natural habitats, over-farming and over-hunting and poaching or simply, human development. Just as prehistoric cultures mixed the fertility of humans with the abundance of the world around them, we are starting to understand the worldwide web of reproductivity, not only among humans but well beyond to other animals, trees, fungi and to entire ecosystems including weather and other atmospheric events, terrestrial and spatial. But we do remain fascinated with the gene as a nexus of control or "life itself," as Sarah Franklin describes it. We hang on to the hope of genetically preserving what we are losing.

We also continue to describe and explain genetically what we can, including recently mothering. Abigail Tucker in her book, *Mom Genes – Inside the New Science of our Ancient Maternal Instinct*, explains how some mammals, humans and a few long-lived whale species stay around to help their daughters mother. Tucker provides ample examples of positive outcomes, physical and mental, for children and their mothers with grandmothers present and helpful, no matter what their socioeconomic backgrounds. In whales where the females continue to live after their reproductivity ends (a rarity among animals, including almost all mammals), they provide maternal direction to the young mothers and food source information to the entire pod that increases the chances of the species' survival, another form of reproduction and another way of understanding survival of the fittest or evolution that relies on mothering. They believe that the primal mother–daughter relationship is etched in our brains. And in 2021 Jennifer Pinkowski reported on recently unearthed evidence that women governed during the prehistoric Bronze Age (3300–1200 BCE).

Another part of the degradation of female reproductivity is the association of menses with failed reproduction and the discarding of unused material, with a similar sense of lack associated with menopause. This attitude has led to the marketing of hormone contraceptive pills so that women experience their period only four times a year as liberating. And as pregnancy and birth were medicalized during the 20th century, menopause stood out for the lack of medical and health attention it garnered. According to the gynaecologist Jen Gunter who published in 2021 *The Menopause Manifesto* on the 200th anniversary of the naming of the term, we are very ill-informed about what menopause is medically and we need to address the stigma associated with it. Gunter describes a "medical silo" where menopause resides today, leaving women in the dark, unable to talk about what is going on in any positive terms and often afraid to approach physicians with their questions or concerns. Post-menopausal women's sexual lives are often considered worthless, and many internalize this.

Gunter's approach differs significantly from previous pharmaceutical ones that aimed to return women to premenopausal hormone levels with hormone replacement therapy (until they found links to hormone sensitive cancers). In the June 6, 2021 issue of *The New York Times*, the reproductive hormone pharmaceutical, Organon, placed a full-page ad proclaiming, "The next big advancement in women's health" over a picture of a giant microphone. Organon is setting itself up as a "new global women's healthcare company" and wants to hear from women everywhere. The hormonal contraceptive market is estimated to reach $20.55 billion by 2026, while as many as 20 million American men at any one time (most of whom are over 50) are reported by David Cox to medicate with Viagra chiefly to reverse impacts of ageing on their sexuality. Pfizer has earned $1.8 billion from Viagra since the early 2000s.

Medical interventions in pregnancy and birth have settled into the political economic and racialized lines that divide populations throughout the world where wealthy, chiefly white women hold the most options to customize their maternity care with very low risks to themselves and their children. Those on the other side of these lines are at much higher risk for prenatal and perinatal issues with spotty to no access to basic healthcare, nutrition and domestic safety and soundness. But all is not over on the medicalization of old reproductive technology: take for example infant formula and breastfeeding. Jenny Kleeman investigates two companies that emerged in 2019 that create artificial human breast milk, one of which, Biomilq, has gained significant investment ($3.5 million) for upscaling operations from the Bill and Melinda Gates Foundation. Biomilq developed a technique to culture mammary cells *in vitro* from cell lines purchased through commercial suppliers for breast cancer research. These cells line the mammary glands and once cultured in the lab start to produce milk, which can be collected. The targeted market includes women who have trouble breastfeeding (physically, psychologically and socially) where the artificial milk is intended to augment the mother's breast milk. They also hope to offer custom-produced milk from the mother's own breast cells. The other company, Singapore's Turtle Tree Labs, uses stem cells to produce and culture mammary cells and plans to license its technology to the world's largest infant formula suppliers. However, no artificial milk can reproduce the capacity of a nursing mother's body to adjust their milk according to ambient temperature (watering it down when more hydration is needed), to fight viral and bacterial infections and to provide the benefits of hormones and bacteria from the mother's biome. What artificial milk addresses are problems associated with using nonhuman milk (intolerances and allergies) as the basis for infant nutrition among the world's wealthy: Turtle Tree Labs estimates it costs them $30 litre to produce artificial human milk. Infant formula promoted in developing countries has long been criticized for masking global economic disparities, placing women and children at risk and providing profits for multinationals.

Meanwhile body-produced breast milk has been found to be an important source of COVID-19 antibodies for newborns, thanks to the quick-thinking doctor and director of a Toronto human milk bank, Sharon Unger. While a wave of Covid patients filled intensive care units, including pregnant women and those who had recently given birth, Unger collected, pasteurized, and stored the breast milk to help these women feed their babies once they recovered. This led to studies of the transmission of the virus through breast milk and to findings that agents in the milk were found to block transmission of the virus through nursing, pasteurization kills the virus and mothers pass on COVID-19 viral antibodies to their nursing infants. Scientists in New York and Israel as well as Toronto are now exploring viral antibody production in breast milk for much broader applications (a new form of wet nursing). Women, especially those vulnerable to the heavy marketing of baby formula in developing countries in the face of restricted water sanitation and nutrition, forgo passing on these protective measures to their infant children as they simultaneously face greater risk of being affected by the virus due to global disparities in basic healthcare provision, including access to vaccines.

Reproducing bodies become a nexus for so much more than reproduction. An important side effect of the medicalization and routinized monitoring of pregnancy has led to the development of a tracking tool for the COVID-19 virus and its variants. Pregnant women's leftover blood samples from public health units across Canada are being examined with the support of the federal COVID-19 Immunity Task Force. They are hoping for a national picture of how the virus and its variants spread across the country. As with Toronto's milk banking story above, this started as an initiative to explore the virus' effect on pregnant women and potential transmission to their infants. Contemporary midwives led by Hannah Dahlen, argued in 2014 that how women give birth (vaginally or by C-section) will eventually change our biomes and genetic makeup due to "wicked" interruptions in what has long been exchanged between mother and newborn. In 2021, the genetic scientist Milissia Maamar and colleagues reviewed the current state of epigenetic inheritance of environmental factors including exposure to DDT on genetic expression over generations of people. Granddaughters of women exposed to DDT run higher genetic propensities to obesity, cardiovascular disease and breast cancer.

An extreme extension of medicalization of reproduction is found in the development of the artificial womb, or ectogenesis, which was used successfully in 2017 to bring a very premature lamb embryo to term by the foetal surgeon, Alan Flake. The transhumanist Zoltan Istvan asks if this can solve the abortion debate. By this he means that any women not wishing to continue with a pregnancy could relinquish the embryo to be brought to term in an artificial womb for prenatal adoption. There is a snag, however: the success with the lamb relied on the embryo being well developed, at the equivalent of about five to six months' human gestation when placed in the artificial womb. Again, technological fixes to social problems appear with little regard for reproductive rights (in this case, the right to early abortion rather than the much more complicated and involved transfer of a five-month embryo), the potential health risks to the developing embryo without the benefit of a pregnant woman and the risks to reproductive justice as decisions are made about which foetuses warrant ectogenesis in the case of extreme premature births. Keep in mind that as late as 2018 Linda Villarosa of *The New York Times* reported that twice as many Black infants in America died as white ones: 4,000 Black infant deaths in a single year. The US remains one of the 13 countries worldwide where the maternal mortality rate is rising, and its Centre for Disease Control reported that the number of preventable near-death events for birthing women between 1993 and 2014 rose 200%, to 50,000 in 2014.

And there are issues within the practice of assisted conception as well. Despite a push for young professional women to rely on NRTs to delay their reproductivity, Sarah Richards of *The New York Times* reported that in 2019 only about 10–14% of women who had frozen and banked their eggs in a NYC area egg bank had come to claim them for reproductive purposes. Many of these women are now beyond reproductive age, and it is presumed they will never return for the eggs. While in 2021 a Rhode Island couple were shocked to find that there were embryos left over from an IVF procedure they underwent over 20 years prior that were still being stored at a fertility centre. They blame a lack of legislation and oversight for stored gametes and embryos slipping through the cracks and not being used as they were intended. They are suing the fertility centre for breach of contract, negligence and intentional infliction of emotional distress.

Genetic engineering is gaining more public exposure and acceptance. A new sort of live genetic engineering museum and lab called Labiomista (meaning the mix of life) opened in Genk in Belgium in July 2019. Oliver Wainwright reports that here are artistic renderings, including taxidermy, of mixed breeds (a pheasant with an iguana's head) along with live animals that the artist Koen Vanmechelen has been breeding for over two decades. He is trying to create the most multicultural and genetically varied chicken in the name of genetic diversity to improve fertility, immunity and resilience. But Vanmechelen has chosen the slow path to genetic engineering; it would be far quicker to genetically engineer the chicken embryos with a tool that is capable of identifying specified genetic strands, cutting them out and replacing them with others with CRISPR-Cas9. Is this critique or preparation for the world to come?

We know CRISPR was used in China to engineer two humans currently alive who have been altered so that they never contact AIDs. We know that the scientific world reacted strongly, claiming this was too much human interference in sex lines too soon. And then the pandemic hit, and we all learned more about viruses with coronas, mRNA vaccines and viral evolution (variants). Jon Gertner of *The New York Times* Sunday Magazine signals this moment as a paradigmatic shift to an acceptance of genomics worldwide. Genomics is the sequencing or detailed description of a genetic code. It requires a large amount of computing power and initially was very expensive. Only one person's entire genetic code was chosen for sequencing, starting October 1990 and completed April 2003. It took a multinational funding and scientific consortium to complete the task which cost over $3 billion. Developments in computing and genetic screening have dropped the cost of genomics by 10 million times and increased the quality 100,000-fold in the last *few years*. The pandemic offered the perfect opportunity for widespread and constant screening of the virus as it spread and mutated, which sent commercial genomics into high gear. The new genomic sequencing machine, Illumina NovaSeq6000 or Nova-*seeks*, was developed from the chiefly publicly funded human gene sequencing project and each machine costs about $1 million (there are 1,000 of them in the world). They can sequence the genes of an entire virus in about two days, and because of a willing Chinese scientist who mounted on the Internet the genetic sequence of a novel virus just identified in Wuhan in January 2020, they have been sequencing COVID-19 from the start. This helped accelerate the development of vaccines and will help with handling the variants. There are also promises for other applications.

By doing widespread genomic sequencing of populations for specific diseases, say Alzheimer's, you can learn a lot about the prevalence of the disease, its uptake, genetic profiles inclined to become diseased and the efficacy (another pandemic term) of treatment. Environmental factors in genetic disease can be uncovered. And PGS could come to mean pre-implantation genomic sequencing – the routine scanning of the entire genomic profile of an individual to map out things like propensities for certain kinds of disease. The social and moral concerns for this are considerable. If you are interested in seeing what they could be, see the film *Gattaca*; it is not as dated as it may seem.

Gertner states how some describe these galloping developments in genetic sequencing and socio-economics as platform technologies. CRISPR-Cas9, used on top of the genomic platform technology, spells out a world of commercial and industrial potential. The researcher Neville Sanjana of the New York Genome Centre uses CRISPR-Cas9, a cheap, quick and easy gene editing tool, to study human disease by modifying and repairing strings of affected DNA. He speaks of the need to continually check his work, which can now be done through cheap, quick and easy genomic technology. Now they are talking in the same breath about "prenatal health," not just screening.

Another potential platform technology in this area is *in vitro* gametogenesis (IVG) or the creation of embryos from egg and sperm cells cultured from stem cells. They have managed this in mice, but the genetic stability in human cells is not certain. As sex cells combine there is always the risk of a genetic slip. Using sex cells that are induced from pluripotent stem cells may increase this risk for a variety of reasons not fully understood in the lab. The implications of clinically applying a technology like this has researchers holding back. For now. The potential for commercial developments from a platform technology like this one, where human genes can be sourced and altered cheaply, quickly and easily, is almost unimaginable.

And then there are the reproductive disruptors. Zoe Beery follows Laurie Bertram Roberts who runs the Mississippi Reproductive Fund helping Black women negotiate the shame-bound and financially prohibitive circuit to abortion in states where TRAP laws reign supreme. She treats her clients with respect and helps to pay bills at home. Same-sex marriage laws have blossomed across the globe over the past decade or so, and there has been increased support for trans people, especially youth, as well as for increasing reproductive rights for LGBTQ2+ communities. These are promising signs of a significant disruption in the reproduction of sexuality (which has implications for our arrangement of sexual reproduction). And there has been serious backlash including the gay club shooting in Orlando, Florida, in 2016, leaving 49 dead and 53 wounded (the US's second largest mass murder) and the brutal and deadly oppression of LGBTQ2+ people in Senegal, Brunei and Russia. It was somewhat hopeful to see that when Andrew Higgins reported on the small Polish town of Krasnik that attempted to keep itself LGBT-free, it drew unwanted global attention as Europe's laughingstock and risked losing EU funding; Krasnik's mayor moved to drop the resolution. And the pandemic left an unexpected drop in already falling birthrates worldwide as well as marked improvements to our natural world. We need to address what reproduction means to us, all of us, to the northern white rhino, to the rain forests of Brazil and to reach far beyond speculations on what's in the test-tube to life as fully lived.

Further reading

Anderson, Sam. 2021. "A mother and daughter at the end." *The New York Times Magazine*, January 10, 22–33, 43, 45.

Beery, Zoe. 2019. "'We are the people we serve'." *The New York Times Magazine*, June 16, 36–39, 51, 53.

Cox, David. 2019. "The race to replace Viagra." *The Guardian Weekly*, June 21, 24–25.

Dahlen, Hannah Grace, Soo Downe, Holly Powell Kennedy, and Maralyn Scotland Foureur. 2014. "Is Society Being Reshaped on a Microbiological and Epigenetic Level By the Way Women Give Birth?" *Midwifery* 30: 1149–1151. DOI: 10.1016/j.midw.2014.07.007.

Franklin, Sarah. 2000. "Life Itself: Global Nature and the Genetic Imaginary." In *Global Nature, Global Culture*, edited by Sarah Franklin, Celia Lury, and Jackie Stacey, 256. London: SAGE.

Gertner, Jon. 2021. "Unlocking the Covid code." *The New York Times*. Accessed 29 May 2021. https://www.nytimes.com/interactive/2021/03/25/magazine/genome-sequencing-covid-variants.html.

Gunter, Jen. 2021. *The Menopause Manifesto: Own Your Health with Facts and Feminism*. Toronto: Penguin Random House.

Higgins, Andrew. 2021. "after voting to be 'free of L.G.B.T.' a polish town pays a price." The *New York Times*, April 11, 9, International.

Istvan, Zoltan 2019. "The artificial womb revolution." *The New York Times*, August 4, 2019.

Kleeman, Jenny. 2020. "'I want to give my child the best': the race to grow human breast milk in a lab." *The Guardian*. Accessed 15 June 2021. https://www.theguardian.com/lifeandstyle/2020/nov/14/i-want-to-give-my-child-the-best-the-race-to-grow-human-breast-milk-in-a-lab.

Maamar, Millissia, Eric Nilsson, and Michael Skinner. 2021. "Epigenetic Transgenerational Inheritance, Gametogenesis and Germline Development." *Biology of Reproduction*: 1–23. DOI: https://doi.org/10.1016/j.pbiomolbio.2012.12.003.

Organon (Advertisement). 2021. "The next big advancement in women's health." *The New York Times*, June 6, 7.

Pinkowski, Jennifer. 2021. "Bronze age tomb hints women helped govern." *The New York Times*, March 14, 14.

Richards, Sarah Elizabeth. 2019. "What happened to all the frozen eggs?" *The New York Times*, December 22, 7, SR.

Rosman, Katherine. 2021. "The lost embryos: a couple's heartbreak." *The New York Times*, June 13, 2021. https://www.nytimes.com/2021/04/16/style/freezing-eggs-and-embryos.html.

Science Daily. 2021. "Oh so simple: eight genes enough to convert mouse stem cells into oocyte-like cells." Accessed 19 June 2021. https://www.sciencedaily.com-releases/2020/12/201216113257.htm.

Subbaraman, Nidhi. 2021. "Lab-Grown Structures Mimic Human Embryo's Earliest Stage Yet." *Nature* 591: 510–511. Accessed 20 June 2021. https://www.nature.com/articles/d41586-021-00695-8.

Tucker, Abigail. 2021. *Mom Genes—Inside the New Science of our Ancient Maternal Instinct*. New York: Gallery Books.

Villarose, Linda. 2018. "The hidden toll." *The New York Times Magazine*, 31–39, 47.

Wainwright, Oliver. 2019. "The stuff of dreams." *The Guardian Weekly*, June 21, 2.

INDEX

For Product Safety Concerns and Information please contact our EU
representative GPSR@taylorandfrancis.com
Taylor & Francis Verlag GmbH, Kaufingerstraße 24, 80331 München, Germany

www.ingramcontent.com/pod-product-compliance
Lightning Source LLC
Chambersburg PA
CBHW060315220326
41598CB00027B/4330